American Medical Association
Physicians dedicated to the health of America

PRACTICE SUCCESS! SERIES

Financial Management of the Medical Practice

The Physician's Handbook for Successful Budgeting, Forecasting & Cost Accounting

Project Manager/Editor: .... Kay Stanley

Project Assistant: .... Kristy Lear

Project Contributors:
Lauretta Mink, CMA, CMM
Max Reibolt, CPA

Art Director: .... Jeff Weir

Published by:

*Coker Publishing Company, LLC —
in affiliation with The Coker Group
3150 Holcomb Bridge Road, Suite 200
Norcross, Georgia 30071
(770) 242-0118*

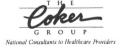

ISBN 0-89970-758-0

American Medical Association Preface _____

This book and others contained in the *PRACTICE SUCCESS!* series are designed to offer you concrete, practical information on topics that you may sometimes consider the least important aspect of the profession of medicine: the business of running a medical practice. And in some ways, that's how it should be. The long, hard years you dedicated to medical school and residency training were meant to make you an excellent physician, not an excellent businessperson. Caring for patients is and always will be your first priority. But you cannot successfully run a medical practice without planning and without consideration of important business issues. While it takes a minimum of ten years for a person to become a physician, the day a practice opens is the day a physician becomes a small businessperson.

Your many years of superb education probably did not include much information on medical office operations, personnel management, accounting or business law. Yet these business issues are more important than ever before, because the practice of medicine in today's rapidly changing environment is far more complex than ever before. Good business management today is essential to good medical practice. The physician who ignores basic business principles in operating his or her practice may soon face difficulties with suppliers, employees, the government or even patients.

Other pressures today force physicians to search for more efficient ways of running their practices. Most physicians find demands on their time increasing tremendously. There is a daily struggle to build a practice that will earn a steady income, to schedule regular working hours, to deliver quality care to patients and to still have time for relaxation and family.

Developing an efficient practice that runs smoothly makes all of these attainable. The application of good business planning will enable you to spend more time on those things that are most important to you.

This book and the others in the *PRACTICE SUCCESS!* series are guides to medical practice management for the new physician and the established physician who wants to survey his or her practice with an eye towards improvement. These books will not provide you with solutions to every challenge that may arise in day-to-day practice. Our goal is to acquaint you with essential business principles and tools, as well as with some new approaches to managing your practice. The knowledge you acquire from this series can be supplemented by information you gather from talking with your colleagues and advisors. You will then be in a position to explore those ideas that promise to achieve the best results for your particular practice situation.

By providing the information in this book and others, the **American Medical Association (AMA)** is not endorsing any one management philosophy or method of delivering health care services. No one approach will meet the objectives of all physicians. Physicians and their staffs will have to decide for themselves what is the best way to manage their individual practices. Finally, this book does not enunciate **AMA** policy. The annual Policy Compendium of the **AMA** sets forth our positions on such issues as contracting, medical ethics, managed care and practice management.

We hope that this publication will be useful to you.

The American Medical Association

About The Coker Group

The Coker Group is a national provider of health care consultative and management services assisting physicians, hospitals, and health care systems to better position themselves to be successful in a reformed health care environment. The Coker Group offers the following services for its clients:

Programs and Services:

- Primary Care Physician Network Development

- Practice Valuations and Acquisition Negotiations

- Physician Employment and Compensation Contract Design

- The Facilitation of Group Practice Development

- Physician Practice Management Services

- Management Services Organization (MSO) Development

- Market Share Management Program

- Newly Recruited Physician Services

- Educational Programs

- Evaluation and Consultant Services

- Personnel Productivity Programs

- *PRACTICE SUCCESS!*© and *PRACTICE SUCCESS!*© Series

For more information, contact:

THE Coker GROUP

National Consultants to Healthcare Providers

The Coker Group / 3150 Holcomb Bridge Road / Suite 200
Norcross, Georgia 30071 / (770) 242-0118

About The Book

Financial Management of the Medical Practice addresses one of the most challenging issues encountered in medical practice management today: how to effectively manage the finances of a medical practice. Because of changes in reimbursement methodology, more than ever before, physician and practice administrators must know how much each procedure costs, and must allocate funds appropriately.

For the non-financial manager, budgeting is often viewed as difficult and tedious. This book is written to dispel the myths about budgeting and forecasting by providing rudimentary exercises in medical practice financial planning. A step-by-step process for budgeting is provided, designed to walk the user through this essential management function.

In addition, this book teaches how to implement guidelines to control cash and establish internal controls covering collections and fraud prevention.

This book is for managers of the business side of medicine.

It is to be used as a guide to understanding the fundamental processes of budgeting, forecasting, and cost accounting. Those who should read it include:

- practicing physicians

- owners of medical practices and clinics

- practice administrators and managers

- business managers of any medical business

- business administrators in health care facilities, nursing homes, or health agencies

Anyone interested in the "how to" aspects of medical practice financial management will benefit greatly from this information. Most physicians have an outside accountant or financial advisor to file tax returns, prepare year-end statements and give general advice and counsel on financial matters. However, it is very important that the physician and practice manager understand sources of revenue and costs of operating the practice. No one can manage what they do not understand and performance cannot be measured unless there are standards in place.

What information can the reader find?

The reader will find practical and specific information and formulas for use in the day-to-day operation of the medical practice, including:

- What is budgeting and forecasting? What do these functions accomplish?

- What is the budgeting process? Who should be involved? What are the major components? What are the outside influences?

- How do I begin? How do I use a budget planning worksheet? How do I forecast patient volume, variable expenses, and revenue? How do I incorporate the budget into the monthly financial statements?

- What do I need to know about cost accounting for the medical practice? What are my sources of revenue? What are the direct and indirect costs, by item and by patient? How do I compile a summary report?

- How do I report operating results?

- How do I understand financial statements and their relationships?

- How do I control overhead?

- How do I establish cash controls? How do I set up controls to reduce the risk of fraud or prevent fraud (omit risk)?

How technical is the writing?

Financial Management of the Medical Practice is written explicitly for the non-financial manager. The title may be a little scary to some but it is mostly a collection of common sense, logical applications interspersed with a measure of good judgment. There are few terms in this book that are not found regularly in a newspaper, and there are no discussions that would appear out-of-place in a business memorandum. This publication is a nontechnical discussion about financial management as it relates to medical practice management.

About the contributors

J. Max Reiboldt, CPA, is Senior Vice President—Finance and Administration of The Coker Group. Mr. Reiboldt is responsible for the company's financial reporting, budgeting, forecasting, review and analysis.   He is also involved in various operational and administrative functions of the company and its overall strategic planning. Mr. Reiboldt helps clients in financial-related matters including negotiation consultations, management services organization (MSO) administration and planning, primary care network development, and practice consultations. He is also a member of the company's Board of Directors.

Mr. Reiboldt has over 23 years of experience in accounting and finance. His background is diversified, with involvement in both the operational and financial functions of a large corporation. He is knowledgeable in human resource management, employee benefits, real estate leasing and development, insurance, and credit and collections.

Mr. Reiboldt performs financial consulting services for health care clients, including medical clinics and privately operated medical laboratories. He routinely completes formal presentations to banks, stockholders, clients, and internal management. In addition, he often speaks at health care conferences, including those sponsored by VHA-Georgia, the National Institute of Physician Recruitment and Retention, and American Health Consultants.

A native of Missouri, Mr. Reiboldt holds a bachelor's degree in accounting from Harding University. He is a member of the American Institute of Certified Public Accountants, and Georgia and Louisiana Societies of CPAs, having also served on various subcommittees.

Lauretta Mink, CMA, CMM, is Vice President—Practice Services of The Coker Group. She has over 27 years of experience in the health care industry. Ms. Mink works extensively with medical practices. Her primary areas of expertise include financial management, practice transition, collection, personnel management, and practice development.

Day-to-day supervision of the management of 20 medical practices has provided her with expert skills in medical management that encompasses budget planning, accounts receivable control, management of overhead, and maintaining a healthy profit margin.

Recently Ms. Mink has been involved with the development and management of an MSO for one of Atlanta's largest hospitals.

Financial Management of the Medical Practice is based on a section excerpt from a 500+ page medical practice management program entitled *PRACTICE SUCCESS!*© Introduced in 1993, this textbook has ongoing updates and enhancements. As publishers, we are committed to providing the most current information covering topics of interest for the "business side of medicine." For more information on this and other resources available, contact:

Coker Publishing Company, LLC
3150 Holcomb Bridge Road
Suite 200
Norcross, GA 30071
(770) 242-0118

Managing Editor
Kay B. Stanley

Overview_____

While there are many more aspects of financial management of the medical practice, this book is an attempt to lay the foundation for improving systems and establishing controls. Budgeting, forecasting, and cost accounting form the basis of financial success in a medical practice. When basic financial principles are ignored, the practice will not achieve its potential—and may ultimately fail.

The information in this book will equip financial decision makers to accomplish these objectives:

- Forecast patient volume, variable and fixed expenses, and revenue.

- Prepare a functional budget to be used to keep the practice financially healthy.

- Understand and control the cost of providing services.

- Manage and control overhead costs of the practice.

- Establish and maintain internal control systems for managing cash and reducing the risk of loss.

- Understand financial statement relationships and reporting procedures.

- Provide a working knowledge of financial terms for non-financial managers.

The forms and exhibits are provided for your use. Duplicate them and use them every day as appropriate. Take time to run the practice well. Whether you practice as a solo practitioner or you are a member of a large group, stay actively involved and informed in the financial affairs of your practice.

Table of Contents

CHAPTER 1

Budgeting and Forecasting

Why Use a Budget?

A budget process is the foundation for all financial activities of the medical practice. It provides and coordinates controls needed to manage the practice effectively.

The managing physician and the practice administrator should understand how to forecast revenues and budget expenses. Practices that have the financial expertise may do budgeting internally. On the other hand, a solo or two-physician practice may choose to have an outside accounting professional conduct these processes.

A budget is generally prepared for a short period (compared to long-range and strategic plans) and is expressed in basic financial terminology. It should be simple enough for the non-accounting professional to understand and to use. Simply stated, a budget measures actual financial performance against standards. A parallel example is to set a personal or professional goal and direct all activities to reach it.

From a practical standpoint, a budget provides an excellent means for understanding the productivity and expense levels that are required to keep the practice financially healthy. The practice administrator who participates in the budget planning exercise benefits professionally by adding a new dimension to his/her skills. By monitoring the actual results versus the budget throughout the year, the practice administrator becomes aware of trends that facilitate better control of future costs. Preparing and monitoring a budget throughout the year (i.e., actual performance versus budgeted standards), provides early warning signs of negative trends within the practice. Budgeting has long been used by businesses in all industries. Traditionally, the medical practice has been financially successful without such a tool. As cost control and other fiscal pressures have developed, now it is necessary for a medical practice to budget like other businesses.

Budgeting is as much a cognitive process as an accounting one. The physician(s) and staff must seriously reflect upon changes in the health care industry and how those changes relate to the practice. Plans for expansion, operational changes concerning services and payor mix, and the physicians' future goals and plans must be considered in the process.

Budgeting includes the coordination, control, and reporting of variances between budgeted and actual results. It relates to all of the policies and procedures needed to accomplish a practice's objectives.

Budgeting Functions/Accomplishments

To summarize, a budget —

- provides an accurate, timely tool to review anticipated versus actual results;

- helps control current performance;

- helps predict future performance and anticipated problem areas;

- determines where resources should be allocated;

- provides an early warning device of budget variations;

- highlights early signs of future opportunities;

- provides the physician(s), office personnel, and practice administrator a practice management tool; and,

- provides a concise financial summary in an understandable format.

The Total Management System

Budgeting entails analysis of all operational and management functions within the practice. It requires *planning* and *action*, followed by constant *review* and *control* considerations. Budgeting involves the following activities:

- determining the initial strategy;

- developing plans to carry out the strategy;

- reflecting the strategic goals and planning process;

- coordinating the organizational structure to fit the goals and strategic plan;

- designing maximization of productivity and revenue;

- developing accurate reporting systems; and,

- developing management control systems with the ability to react and respond to variances.

The budgeting process is a small, but very important, link in the chain in the practice management cycle. For such a continuum of processes, none of the components (i.e., links in the chain) can break down. Budgeting, forecasting, and cost allocation are vital to a healthy, successful management system.

The Budgeting Process

Who Should Be Involved?

The budgeting process starts with a budget planning session. All key decision makers and other personnel in cost containment roles must attend. Those participating should include:

- Physician(s);

- Practice administrator;

- Department heads, if applicable.

The following information should be compiled prior to the meeting to be used as resource material for formulation of the initial budget. Once this information has been collected, plan on a three-hour session.

- Year-end financial statements for the prior three fiscal periods, preferably broken down by month or at the very least, by quarter. Depending on the legal structure of the practice, tax returns may also be beneficial.

- All legal documents supporting contractual agreements. These include real estate leases, equipment leases, contracts for cleaning, maintenance, landscaping, etc.

- List of major equipment purchases anticipated for the coming year, including the estimated cost and suggested method of payment for each. Consider all possible acquisitions regardless of the cost impact on the practice (i.e., a "wish list" of items).

- Fee schedules.

- All productivity reports or practice analyses generated by the practice management software system. These include analysis by physician of overall production versus collections, payor mix, utilization information, etc.

- A list of planned new services for the coming year. In consultation with the physician(s), this should be determined and incorporated in the budgeting process.

- List of outside influences that may directly affect the practice (e.g., specific industry issues, managed care contracting changes, political issues, demographic considerations, technological matters, and general business considerations).

Outside Influences on the Budgeting Process

The medical practice has been somewhat insulated from the phenomenon of outside influences on the budgeting process. As changes occur in the environment of governmental agencies and private outside payors (such as insurance companies), the influences of the outside world on a medical practice increase. Hence, the following economic factors must be considered in the budgeting process:

- Inflation rates;

- Anticipated interest or cost of capital rates;

- Labor costs;

- Regulatory influences and requirements;

- Material and supply costs, including office and medical supplies;

- Competition considerations directly affecting the practice;

- Demographic considerations, including possible changes;

- Products and services being offered within the practice; and,

- Potential changes to other health care providers that will affect the practice (e.g., hospital mergers, HMO acquisitions, etc.).

Budgeting — How To Begin

Major Components of the Budget Planning Worksheet

The Budget Planning Worksheet is a critical tool in the budget planning process. To use it efficiently, we must have a clear understanding of the major types of revenue and expenses.

- **Gross Revenue**

  Generally refers to all production placed "on the books" by the physician for services rendered. This includes such items as office visits, consultations, hospital visits and procedures, ancillary procedures, nursing home work, and outpatient procedures.

- **Contractual Adjustments to Revenue**

  The resulting discount applied to gross revenue (e.g., that generated from Medicare and Medicaid price reductions and managed care discounts on both a fee-for-service and a capitated basis).

- **Fee-for-Service Revenue**

  That revenue produced for the physician as a result of the specific service performed. No consideration is made for number of patients seen or any other outside influence other than actually considering the fee to be charged for that specific service.

- **Capitated Income**

  Income tied to a number of "covered lives" subject to a managed care contract in which a guaranteed payment rate per covered life is paid to the physician, regardless of whether the patient subject to the contract is seen by the physician.

- **Net Collections**

  Since most practices are accounted for on a "cash basis," this is the "actual revenue" referred to for the budget planning process. It represents the actual receipts of the practice, net of all contractuals, and is a result of the actual collections of accounts receivable from all sources of professional services performed by the physician. The net collections total, therefore, is the most critical item of the revenue side of the budget planning process upon which decisions are to be based.

- **Fixed Expenses**

  Expenses not affected by patient volume. Examples are rent, salaries (excluding commissions), interest payments on fixed debt, insurance, property taxes, and utilities.

- **Variable Expenses**

  Expenses that change in direct proportion to the number of patients seen. Examples are medical supplies, office supplies, laboratory costs, medications, and interest on an operating working capital line of credit.

- **Period Expenses**

  Costs incurred over time as opposed to level of activity. As an example, salaries are quoted as an annual amount, but paid over a period of time during the year.

Developing the Budget Planning Worksheet

The Budget Planning Worksheet provides a basis to formulate the financially compiled information. Briefly, let's review the key contents of this simple worksheet (see Exhibit 1-1-1).

- **Items**

  These represent typical revenue and expense accounts to be considered in a budgeting process. While there is no "all inclusive list," those listed on Exhibits 1-1-1 and 1-1-2 are typical practice revenue and expense accounts. Prepare your list to fit the needs of your practice.

  For this worksheet, revenues represents *net collections* from the practice. For purposes of this exercise, do not include gross production in revenues prior to contractual adjustments and/or discounts. Rather, net collections represent the final, anticipated collections total, net of all such contractual adjustments and discounts.

  Expense items include broad accounts such as accounting, contributions, insurance, supplies, rent, salaries, taxes, depreciation, etc. Again, these items should be specific to your practice needs.

- **1993–1994**

  The 1993–1994 columns represent the previous two years (assuming this is a 1996 budget). These are the actual operating results for each of the items listed for these years.

- **Percentage Change**

  This column represents the difference between 1993 and 1994 actual performance for each line item. To calculate the percentage, subtract 1994 actual total from 1993 actual total for a line item and divide the difference by the 1993 total. Reflect the calculated amount as a percentage in this column.

- **1995**

  This represents the actual totals for each item for the most recent year, 1995.

- **Percentage Change**

  This is the difference between 1995 and 1994 actual results calculated as a percentage. The computation is similar to that noted previously in the first Percentage Change column.

- **Initial Budget**

  This amount is the first item entered on the worksheet for projected totals. Its input is without the benefit of detailed analysis and consideration on the part of the physician(s) and practice administrator. In other words, it is the initial "pass" at the numbers based upon prior years results.

- **Final Budget**

  These totals are the result of much deliberation, analyses and consideration of the numbers. They relate to the actual operations of the practice. Final budget numbers reflect adjustments made from the Initial Budget to meet certain goals and objectives of the practice. They also reflect realities that exist for expenses to be controlled and revenues to be realized.

- **Percent of Revenue**

  This column represents the final budgeted total for each expense item as a percent to the total net collections of revenue (i.e., net collections).

At the bottom of the Budget Planning Worksheet are two totaling lines. The first is *Total* for *Expenses.* This simply adds each of the expense items for each particular column. The final line is *Net Income Prior to Physician Compensation.* This is the difference between the total net collections and total expenses for each column. **In all instances, the Budget Planning Worksheet is prior to any consideration for any physician compensation. This is regardless of whether or not physicians are operating on a guaranteed income as an employee or completely independent. And if independent, it is also prior to any consideration of any guaranteed wage or monthly draw for physician compensation.**

Beginning the Budget Planning Worksheet

In order to begin the *Budget Planning Worksheet,* complete the columns that require actual information.

- Completing the budget requires both detail analysis and planning. For each line item on the budget, look at previous financial reports for amounts historically spent. Be careful not to assume that just because we have always spent $500 per year for magazines, newspapers and publications that it is a necessary expenditure. This is where the planning comes in: What is the value of this expense? Who reads the materials? What would happen if we cut the expense to $100 per year?

- Enter all the titles of expense categories under the *Items* column of the *Budget Planning Worksheet.*

- Enter the actual dollar amount spent in each of the last three years.

- Calculate the percent of change for each item for each year and enter this percent into the Percent *Change* column.

- Apply the percent of change to last year's dollar amount and enter the dollar figure in the *Initial Budget* column. (Remember, this is simply a calculated amount based upon prior years' actual results and trends and is only used as a start from which to complete the detailed analysis to formulate the *Final Budget* figure.)

The result of these calculations is an *unadjusted* budget figure for revenue (i.e., *net collections*) and each expense for the coming year.

Completing the Final Budget

More detailed analysis and planning is required to complete the final budgeted totals. Review each expense line (i.e., both historical results and future projections). Consider expenses and revenues in broad terms such as patient comfort, employee job enrichment, etc. Relate these to specific expenses to help to understand how this final budget is determined.

First, let's look at *Fixed Expenses* (those not affected by patient volume). On the Budget Planning Worksheet, enter the actual dollar amount spent during the previous three years; calculate the *Percent Change*; enter in the *Initial Budget* column the actual expense from the actual percentage change for the most recent year applied to that year's actual amount. Or, if you know of a contractual change (such as a new janitorial contract) occuring that will affect a different monthly and annual charge from previous expenses, enter that total.

Example: If salaries were $165,900 in 1993; $171,800 in 1994; and, $175,900 in 1995, you have experienced a 3.4 percent increase from 1994 versus 1993 and a 2.4 percent increase from 1995 versus 1994. Obviously, the most recent year's increase of 2.4 percent holds more weight than the previous year's 3.4 percent in deriving the Initial Budget total versus an

average of the two years. Thus, use the most recent year's increase, assuming that trend will continue. With that assumption, the Initial Budget total for 1995 for salaries is $180,100. Post this amount in the Initial Budget column.

The result of completing the calculations for all Fixed Expenses is an *unadjusted* or Initial Budget total for those items.

Budget Planning Worksheet

Exhibit 1-1-1

Items	1993	1994	% Change	1995	% Change	Initial Budget	Final Budget	% of Revenue
Revenue "Net Collections"*								
Accounting/Legal								
Contributions								
Dues/Subscriptions								
Equipment Rental								
General Insurance								
Health Insurance								
Malpractice Insurance								
Lab Fees								
Janitorial								
Medical Supplies								
Office Supplies								
Rent or Lease								
Salaries								
Taxes-Payroll								
Taxes-Other								
Telephone								
Postage								
Maintenance, Repairs								
Interest								
Depreciation								
Professional Services								
Profit Sharing								
Other								
Total Expenses								
Net Income Pre-Physician Comp.								

*Note: "Net Collections" represent the actual monies received and deposited into the practice. It considers the effect of discounts and contractual adjustments or write-offs from gross billings. It would include: *Billings or Gross Charges Less Discounts, Gross Revenue Less Write-offs, Revenue, Net Collections.*

Budget Planning Worksheet

Exhibit 1-1-2

Items	1993	1994	% Change	1995	% Change	Initial Budget	Final Budget	% of Revenue
Revenue "Net Collections"	856,900	881,600	2.8%	886,000	0.5%	928,943	915,000	100.0%
Accounting/Legal	8,000	5,800	-37.9%	5,400	-6.9%	5,400	5,400	0.6%
Contributions	2,500	5,000	50.0%	600	-88.0%	600	1,000	0.1%
Dues/Subscriptions	2,000	2,500	20.0%	2,000	-20.0%	2,000	2,000	0.2%
Equipment Rental	0	0	0.0%	15,500	0.0%	15,000	15,000	1.6%
General Insurance	46,800	47,300	1.1%	49,800	5.3%	50,000	51,000	5.6%
Health Insurance	33,600	18,100	-85.6%	9,800	-45.9%	10,200	10,200	1.1%
Malpractice Insurance	15,900	20,400	22.1%	19,700	-3.4%	20,500	20,500	2.2%
Lab Fees	97,500	133,100	26.7%	124,000	-6.8%	126,548	127,000	13.9%
Janitorial	1,500	1,600	6.3%	1,600	0.0%	1,600	1,600	0.2%
Medical Supplies	15,400	17,800	13.5%	10,600	-40.4%	10,880	11,000	1.2%
Office Supplies	29,300	28,800	-1.7%	8,500	-70.5%	8,738	8,800	1.0%
Rent or Lease	49,700	49,100	-1.2%	44,100	-10.2%	49,700	49,700	5.4%
Salaries	165,900	171,800	3.4%	175,900	2.4%	180,100	180,000	19.7%
Taxes-Payroll	32,100	33,200	3.3%	31,900	-3.9%	33,000	33,000	3.6%
Taxes-Other	2,200	4,700	53.2%	7,500	59.6%	8,000	8,000	0.9%
Telephone	22,500	24,700	8.9%	22,600	-8.5%	23,120	23,000	2.5%
Postage	5,300	7,700	31.2%	7,700	0.0%	7,922	8,000	0.9%
Maintenance, Repairs	4,800	4,900	2.0%	5,500	12.2%	6,000	6,000	0.7%
Interest	7,300	5,100	-43.1%	4,900	-3.9%	4,500	4,500	0.5%
Depreciation	7,500	8,400	10.7%	8,000	-4.8%	8,000	8,000	0.9%
Professional Services	9,400	16,700	43.7%	10,000	-40.1%	10,500	10,500	1.1%
Profit Sharing	16,700	1,000	-1570.0%	1,800	80.0%	1,900	1,900	0.2%
Other	800	1,600	50.0%	15,500	868.8%	10,000	5,000	0.5%
Total Expenses	**576,700**	**609,300**	**5.4%**	**579,900**	**-4.8%**	**593,708**	**591,100**	**64.6%**
Net Income Pre-Physician Comp.	**280,200**	**272,300**	**-2.9%**	**306,100**	**0.3%**	**335,235**	**323,900**	**35.4%**

Forecasting Patient Volume

Before Variable Expenses (those that change with patient volume) can be accurately projected, you must first determine how *Patient Volume* will change. Hence, before resuming our analysis of the Budget Planning Worksheet and Variable Expenses, we will consider *Patient Volume*.

To establish a basis to forecast *Patient Volume*, answer the following questions:

- What patient volume trends have developed over the past three years? Is the average percent of change in patient volume for the past two years expected to continue?

- Will there be any significant changes in managed care contracting that will result in an increase, decrease, or discontinuation of contracts resulting in less volume?

- Will the practice add a physician extender (e.g., Physician Assistant or Nurse Practitioner) to the practice? If so, what potential impact will this have on the patient volume?

- Does the practice plan to discontinue a service (i.e., obstetrical care) that could decrease patient volume? Conversely, are there services that can be added to the practice that will increase patient volume?

- How many hours per day and how many days per week will the physician(s) conduct their office practice?

- What does competition dictate as far as the particular specialty of the practice? Have additional physicians in your specialty moved into the market area presenting new competition?

- What is the marketing plan to promote the practice for the coming year? A more aggressive marketing approach should increase volume. Obviously, the cost versus the projected volume increase must be weighed.

- How far out are you giving appointments to a patient. If the wait seems unreasonable to the patient (for a non-emergency call), you should expect patients to look for another physician. Here is where you may consider either hiring a PA or NP or extending your practice hours.

To illustrate the above, assume the following about your practice and its competition:

- Your practice is well-established in the community and you have a high level of recognition and credibility. Managed care has increased your patient base by 300 covered lives through your first HMO contract. From your discussions with the HMO, you anticipate an addition of eight patients per month to the practice.

- Your patient volume has remained essentially constant over the past three years outside of the increased managed care business, and no appreciable increase in patient volume is expected for 1996.

- A new physician in your specialty has just been recruited to the community and will set up practice less than ten miles from yours. From all indications, this practice could pull away some of your patients, if for no other reason than geographical proximity.

This illustration of forecasting patient volume is simple and factored on a easily determined set of circumstances. However, give careful consideration to the entire market area to determine any other factors that will affect patient volume.

Continuing with this example, based upon your research, use the historical results of a flat patient volume variance over the past three years along with the increased managed care business. We will assume that the managed care contract will be a fee-for-service (non-capitated) contract. With capitation, the revenues from this contract may actually be easier to project than otherwise. Again, we assume that based on practice history there will be no increase in patient volume. However, through managed care we can project eight new patients per month (96 per year). Based on a projected $100 per patient average fee, the result is an increased revenue of $800 per month ($9,600 per year).

Also consider that you may lose as many as ten patients per month to the new physician during the first six months. You estimate that this will level off during the last six months of the year to no more than three patients per month. Therefore, forecast your patient attrition (loss) at six patients per month or 72 per year. Thus, you estimate a loss of 72 visits and a gain of 96 visits for *a net gain of 24 patient visits for the year.*

With the flat projection for standard patient volume, your overall projected increase in patient visits in the coming year is 24. If we chart this based on patient visits alone, the result is a small net increase in patient visits for the coming year.

This is merely one example of how such a forecast can be completed and quantified. This total is then converted into a dollar amount to derive total patient volume for the year. This must then be converted based upon contractual obligations and write-offs in order to derive a *net collected cash total* upon which the Budget Planning Worksheet is based.

In summary, many factors affect the number of patients seen. The practice cannot assume that patient volume will increase every year. Remember, in our example we actually assumed no increase before other new factors were considered (i.e., the new managed care contract and the new practice). The more aware the practice is of what is going on in its market area and the industry in general, the more accurately it can forecast changes.

The real benefit of a well-planned practice budget comes from careful consideration of changes and the ability to accurately reflect or forecast these upon the practice operations.

Forecasting Variable Expenses

Having illustrated how to forecast Patient Volume, we can more accurately forecast the expenses that will change with that volume. The first step to determining and forecasting *Variable Expenses* is to calculate the current cost per patient. To accomplish this, refer to Exhibit 1-2-1 and Exhibit 1-2-2, *Patient Cost Analysis*. Exhibit 1-2-2 indicates the appropriate entries and calculations to derive a revenue per patient total.

Patient Cost Analysis   Exhibit 1-2-1

1. Total number of patients seen for prior 12 months .... _____

2. Total of all expenses for prior 12 months .... _____

3. Subtract from line 2 all **Fixed Expenses** (rent, salaries and benefits, insurance, utilities) .... _____

4. Total **Patient** expenses for prior 12 months .... _____

5. Total receipts for prior 12 months .... _____

6. Divide line 5 by line 1 to get gross revenue per patient .... _____

7. Divide line 4 by line 1 to get cost per patient .... _____

8. Subtract line 7 from line 6 to get revenue per patient .... _____

Patient Cost Analysis Example

Exhibit 1-2-2

1. Total number of patients seen for prior 12 months 15,600

2. Total of all expenses for prior 12 months $579,000.00

3. Subtract from line 2 all **Fixed Expenses** (rent, salaries
    and benefits, insurance, utilities) $360,100.00

4. Total **Patient** expenses for prior 12 months $219,800.00

5. Total receipts for prior 12 months...$886,000.00

6. Divide line 5 by line 1 to get gross revenue per patient...$56.79

7. Divide line 4 by line 1 to get cost per patient $14.09

8. Subtract line 7 from line 6 to get revenue per patient..$42.70

Let's review each line item of this example:

Line Number 1 - Total Number of Patients Seen for Prior Twelve Months

This should be the actual office visits recorded by the physician(s). Unless you are performing these projections at the end of your current fiscal period, it would be more accurate to use the last twelve months' data.

Line Number 2 - Total of All Expenses for the Prior Twelve Months

This is an entry directly off your financial statements. It should not include compensation to the physician(s).

Line Number 3 - Fixed Expenses

Fixed Expenses such as rent, salaries, insurance, and utilities should be subtracted from Line Number 2 to derive this entry.

Line Number 4 - Total Patient Expenses.

Line Number 5- Actual Cash Receipts for the Prior Twelve Months.

Line Number 6 - Gross Revenue Per Patient is calculated by dividing Line Number 5 by Line Number 1. In our example, the $56.79 total revenue per patient is calculated.

Line Number 7 - Cost Per Patient is calculated by dividing Line Number 4, Total Patient Expenses by Line Number 1, Total of Number Patients Seen for Prior Twelve Months.

Line Number 8- Net Revenue Per Patient is the subtraction of Line Number 7 from Line Number 6.

Before we complete our review of **Forecasting Variable Expenses,** let's consider **Forecasting Revenue.**

Forecasting Revenue

We already learned that determining patient volume is the first step in forecasting revenue. We considered both internal and external changes anticipated within the practice to develop a logical projection of patient visits for the coming year.

Another component in forecasting revenue is to determine if and how much of an increase in the fee schedule the practice plans to make. We recommend that, at the very least, a practice adjust its fees at the beginning of each year. This can be accomplished by two simple methods:

- Applying a percent of increase to every fee based upon inflation, an inflation index, or a cost of living change or specific factors in the individual practice which ultimately dictate an adjustment.

- Reviewing each fee and increasing those that have increased in cost to deliver.

A knowledge of one's costs is a significant component of successfully negotiating and securing a managed care contract. A fee schedule can literally be dictated based upon such contracting. While differences in fee schedules may exist depending upon the payor (e.g., indemnity insurance versus Medicare versus HMO or PPO managed care), it is best to have a consistent fee schedule and not change it to accommodate the different types of payors. However, as software is improved for managed care, it will allow the user to input many different fee schedules for each managed care plan. The system will enter the proper fee initially so no adjustments will need to be made.

Competition is another factor to consider when making a change in the fee schedule. It is helpful to know what your competition is charging for comparable services. Remember, it is acceptable to "shop" competitive prices, but it is probably illegal for practices to agree to a uniform pricing schedule.

Though it may be difficult to anticipate the effect of a fee schedule change in the budget planning process, an easy and safe approach is to apply a two percent or three percent cost of living adjustment for inflation. Remember, the preparation of a budget is primarily for internal use and requires you to be conservative and realistic. If a fee schedule is increased by more than a simple cost of living adjustment and that increase is a certainty, reflect that in the budget. However, if it is not a certainty, particularly when completing the Budget Planning Worksheet, then a simple increase may be justified. On the other hand, if managed care contracting will result in lowering the fee schedule, then this should be realistically reflected in the projections.

Another step in forecasting revenue is to determine if the practice plans to offer new services to generate additional revenue. An example might be the purchase of a flexible sigmoidoscope in order to perform flexible sigmoidoscopies in the office. To accurately project revenues a new service might generate, some historical information will be needed. If it is not available, then realistic projections must be used. For example, historical information might tell you that the practice performed 100 sigmoidoscopies last year and referred another 50 patients to the outpatient gastroenterology center at the hospital, etc.

You could project that you will do 100 sigmoidoscopies next year based on 300 complete physical examinations given last year; you assume that at least one in three of those would need a sigmoidoscopy as a screening procedure.

The average fee for *CPT Code 45330 Sigmoidoscopy Flexible Fiber Optic Diagnostic* is more than $50. You project doing 100 Sigmoidoscopies at $150 for an estimated $15,000 in additional revenue.

Your projections determine that revenues will increase at a three percent inflation rate over the prior year due to an across-the-board fee schedule increase. Thus, three percent of the estimated $886,000 base revenue results in $26,580 additional revenue for the new year.

Add to this figure the revenue you would gain from the increased patient volume projected earlier, (i.e., 24 new patients X $56.79 or $1,362.96 in additional revenue). Note: The $56.79 revenue per patient is a result of our previous calculation of gross revenue per patient completed in Exhibit 1-2-2, *Patient Cost Analysis.*

Altogether the three increases will provide $42,942.96 in added revenues to be budgeted in the next year:

Added Services	$15,000.00
Fee Increases	26,580.00
New Patients	1,362.96
Total	**$42,942.96**

This amount is reflected in the Budget Planning Worksheet, *Initial Budget* column.

Now that we have reviewed forecasting patient volume, let's resume our consideration of *Variable Expenses* (those that change with patient volume and can be projected in a step-by-step process).

Step One is to determine the level of cost increase expected for each of the Variable Expenses. For example, ask yourself the question, "What was the average percent of increase for medical supplies over the last three years?" Refer to your Budget Planning Worksheet (Exhibits 1-1-1 and 1-1-2) for this entry. A sensible follow-up question would be, "Is it reasonable to expect the cost of supplies in the coming year will increase as much as the average increase over the past three years?" If the answer to this question is yes, then the inclusion of the average percentage increase over last year's actual figure to develop next year's Initial Budget total is appropriate.

In our example we forecasted a slight increase in Patient Volume. In doing this, an obvious increase in the cost of seeing patients must be considered. The simplest method is to take the cost per patient calculated for each patient last year on the Patient Cost Analysis Worksheet (see Exhibit 1-2-2) and multiply this dollar amount by the projected net gain of patients. For example, earlier we projected a net gain of 24 patients for the new year. In Exhibit 1-2-2, we calculated the prior year's average cost per patient as $14.09. Multiply the 24 patients by $14.09 to determine a total cost of $338 to see these additional patients.

Next, determine the number of Variable Expense categories. If there are five, divide the total reached in the above calculation by five and enter an equal amount of the increase to each of these five expense categories. For example, let's assume that the only Variable Expenses are office supplies, medical supplies, laboratory expenses, x-ray expenses, and transcription fees; and, because of their nature, they all change with patient volume. In this exercise, $338 divided by 5 equals $67.60. Add $68 to each of the five expense categories. The amounts vary according to the number of Variable Expenses categories.

To complete the Budget Planning Worksheet Initial Budget column, convert to dollars the percent of increase you have determined for each Variable Expense. For example, medical supply costs have increased an average of two percent over the last three years. Assume that you will experience the same level of increase next year. Medical supply costs last year were $10,600, so increase this figure by two percent, or to $10,812. Add to this the $68, the determined cost for medical supplies to see the additional 24 patients. The total budgeted amount for medical supplies is $10,880.

Final Budget Column Entries

Having completed all of the calculations and input for the Initial Budget column, we now have a good start toward the Final Budget figure. Before proceeding, take time to consider all other factors within the practice that will influence the Final Budget total. Such factors might include a realistic overview of what is going on within the practice or the knowledge of an external or internal factor that will significantly change the initial budgeted total to the final entry. The key decision makers should review each line entry to assist in the formulation of the Final Budget. **Remember, regardless of how well analyzed and thought through a budget might be, it requires a total buy-in of the physician(s) and/or other owners of the practice in order to be taken seriously and result in the useful management tool it is intended to be.**

The Final Step

Now that you have arrived at a realistic budget figure for each projected expense and the operating revenues, the final step is to calculate the percent of each expense to total revenue projected. Interpreting all budgeted data, especially expense entries on a line-by-line basis, is very important. Converting expenses as a percent of total net collections is essential. Many of the industry published guidelines are only reflected as a percent of collections. For example, a practice which operates at a 50 percent or less expense factor (i.e., 50 percent of net collections for total expenses, excluding physician compensation) is generally looked upon to have a fairly efficient structure. Conversely, when a budget is prepared resulting in an expense total in excess of 50 percent, further research will be needed in order to ascertain if this will be acceptable. Historically, if a practice has operated on a 55 percent or 60 percent of net collections expense factor, the physician(s) and/or other owners of the practice may find this acceptable. While not an acceptable industry standard, if the owners don't object, the final budget may reflect such a high expense total.

Remember, expense to earnings percentages do vary with geographical locations, the specialty, and the type of practice, such as solo versus group. The benchmark figures for your specialty are available from several sources (i.e., the American Medical Association, Medical Group Management Association, or local consulting firms). In addition, *Medical Economics* publishes these expense averages each year in its November issue.

Thus, the final step of calculating the percentages of each expense item to total net collections is a process which brings the budgeted figures into perspective.

The Reality Check

The outcome of completing of the Budget Planning Worksheet is a true internal assessment. In other words, *The Reality Check.*

After the budget has been set and final entries have been completed, the practice administrator and physician(s) should look at the totals on an overall basis. Previously, we discussed the percentages of expense items to net collections as a ongoing process throughout the formulation of the budget and should not necessarily be delayed until the budget is complete. On the other hand, when all of the numbers are entered and the calculations made with the totals set for the budget, it is logical and somewhat easier to take this overall look at what has been done and incorporate it into the reality of running the practice.

The Reality Check, should ask the following questions for each entry:

- Is this entry realistic?

- Can we afford the increases or decreases?

- Will the increases maintain the practice at a competitive level and result in efficient operation comparable to prior years?

- What does management, usually the physician(s), really want?

Another part of *The Reality Check* is to analyze if the expenses are reasonable in light of where the practice is going and what has traditionally been acceptable performance. Physicians are sometimes more interested in maintaining a certain level of quality or prestige in their practice than concerned about the costs to maintain these. For example, certain practice commodities are not necessary, such as providing a coffee service, bottled water, etc. If a practice is under pressure to cut expenses, logically these would be the first areas to cut. However, before cutting or eliminating these expenses, the physician(s) must be consulted and clearly agree to the cuts. On the other hand, it would not be fair to cut the budget for such items with no real intention of actually putting them into action.

Part of *The Reality Check* is therefore converting the numbers to the real life of running the day-to-day practice. A budget is not useful nor beneficial if it does not reflect the actual day-to-day occurrences and expense considerations. Therefore, the linking of numbers on a piece of paper that ultimately is called the "Budget" with the actual realities of the practice's operations is essential. Sometimes the reluctance to complete this linking causes the entire budgeting process to be useless.

Incorporating the Budget Into the Monthly Income Statement

When you are satisfied that your budget figures are as accurate and as realistic as possible, ask your accounting professional or write-up firm to add these figures to your *Monthly Income Statement*. Then each month you will have a comparison of the actual figures to the budgeted amounts. A sample *Income Statement* with columns for budget and variance is provided in Exhibit 1-3.

Monthly monitoring of the actual operating results with the budgeted figures is therefore an essential process. This becomes a *working budget,* not one that is simply placed on a shelf or in a drawer after it is completed with no further consideration.

If you see monthly actual results that are considerably higher or lower than the budgeted figures, do not over-react, but research the variances to determine why they occurred. Closely monitor the results at least for a couple of months to determine real trends. Frequently you will see leveling out over the course of the year. Remember that a budget that is done correctly is a useful management tool that gives early detection of either negative or positive trends. Do not wait too long to bring such variances to the attention of the physician(s) and be prepared to satisfactorily present the reasons for the variances. Complete a summary to supplement the monthly financial statements given to the physician(s) that explain the significant variances. Regardless, the key is to always research monthly overages or shortages to see why such an unexpected result has occurred.

When the budgeted totals are prepared with care and forethought (therefore, realistic and accurate), their comparison to actual results bears more analytical weight than comparisons with actual prior year's totals. After the process is completed and incorporated into the financial statement process, it forms the basis of future decision making.

Physicians are facing dramatic health care reform and this will continue to be the case for the next few years. It is now necessary to operate more cost effectively. The increasing pressure to discount fees for large blocks of patients is expected to continue. Increasing the physicians' income, as well as limiting expenses, will be more important than ever before to the operation and management of a medical practice. In the "good ole days" generally a medical practice provided an excellent income. Physicians were well compensated without having to plan or budget. Those days are over. Physicians must now understand what it takes to operate a practice *profitably*. Planning, which is formalized in budget, helps produce a successful and profitable practice.

In short, the successful medical practice of the 1990s will identify and react to the impact of outside economic factors and *plan* its internal operations accordingly.

Income Statement   Exhibit 1-3

	Current Month			Year-to-date		
	Budget	**Actual**	**% Variance**	**Budget**	**Actual**	**% Variance**
Income						
Charges						
Other Adjustments						
Other Receipts						
Total Income						
Expenses						
Salaries – Office						
Answering Service and Pager						
Automobile						
Consultant Fees						
Conventions and Meetings						
Contributions						
Depreciation						
Dues/Subscriptions						
Employee Benefits						
Gifts/Flowers						
Insurance – Business						

	Current Month			Year-to-date		
	Budget	Actual	% Variance	Budget	Actual	% Variance
Insurance – Malpractice						
Laundry – Uniforms						
Legal & Accounting						
Medical Pamphlets & Books						
Miscellaneous						
Office Supplies & Expense						
Postage						
Profit Sharing						
Rent						
Repairs & Maintenance						
Supplies – Medical						
Taxes & Licenses						
Telephone						
Transcription Fees						
X-Ray Expense						
Total Expenses						
Operating Income <Loss>						

CHAPTER 2

Revenue and Cost Accounting

Just as documentation of revenues and expenses is necessary for tax reporting purposes, it is as equally important and necessary to efficiently manage the medical practice. In previous chapters, we discussed how important the budgeting process is in controlling the *direction* of the practice. Now we will consider ways to track certain *revenue and expense* items by *sources.* Further, we will review proper methods of cost allocation analysis. It is crucial in today's health care environment that practice management knows and understands the costs to deliver its professional services. Allocations of overhead to cost or profit centers within the practice result in meaningful information that will assist the practice administrator and physician(s) in determining the direction of the practice.

Sources of Revenue

The first step is to track the sources of revenue within the practice. This step enables the practice administrator and physician(s) to identify the most profitable areas of revenue production and also helps track the cause of lost revenue.

Within every medical practice, revenue is generated through specific production and revenue centers. The most common are:

- Medical (Patient Visits)
- Surgical
- Laboratory
- Radiology
- Endoscopy
- Pharmacy

Determining the costs and revenue generated by each revenue center will provide necessary information for financial planning. Revenue centers are easy to segregate by type of service performed. In looking at sources of revenue, particularly as they relate to managed care contracting, we need to determine the services that generate the greatest and most profitable levels of production. For example, based upon our analysis of both the ability to produce revenue and the costs to produce it (costs will be analyzed in subsequent sections of this chapter), we should be able to determine the areas of production (i.e., revenue centers) that should be emphasized. As an example, we may determine that the best and most profitable source of revenue for a Family Practitioner is office inpatient visits. This being true, then one strategy for this practice could be to increase the physician's office time. Conversely, if it is determined that rendering laboratory services are not profitable, or at least as profitable, then very little time or investment should be placed in providing laboratory services.

In manufacturing, a company typically makes several products. Each product has a separate accounting with costs allocated accordingly. The cost accounting for a particular product in a manufacturing setting will be performed in a way to fairly depict the profit margin for each product.

A medical practice may use a similar approach. Financial statements may be prepared by revenue center with proper allocations of certain "corporate" or practice overhead. Expense items such as salaries, rent, specific supply items, benefits, etc., should be included. While our discussion in earlier chapters on budgeting did not illustrate the budgeting process by revenue center, this process can easily be adapted to budgeting, as well. However, many revenue centers exist as separate budgets with one consolidated budget reflecting the entire practice (i.e., individual budgets added together to make the total). It is essential to know the potential revenue and costs within a particular service or component of the practice.

Cost Analysis by Revenue Center

The knowledge of one's costs within a medical practice for each of the revenue centers is absolutely essential to successfully negotiate a managed care contract. However, no matter what the environment, whether a standard, fee-for-service or a heavy managed care environment, this information is indispensable. A computerized practice management program will provide a productivity analysis by revenue center.

To control costs — a necessary requirement of running a practice today — they must be identified by department or revenue center. In a large practice or medical clinic, each physician or specialty may be considered a revenue center, as may each ancillary department (such as laboratory and radiology). There are two types of costs that should be determined for each revenue center, *direct* and *indirect*. The following gives an example of each of these costs as they relate to a Radiology Department within the practice:

Direct Costs

The following are considered costs specifically associated with the Radiology Department. In other words, if the Radiology Department does not exist, neither do these costs:

- Film
- Maintenance and Repair to X-ray Equipment
- Developer and Fixer
- Technician's Salary
- Fees for Radiologist's review, if applicable

Indirect Costs

Indirect costs are those that are not specifically associated with a department and would not be eliminated if the service were not offered. The following are typical examples of indirect costs:

- That percentage of leased spaced occupied by the X-ray room
- Utilities
- Additional expenses such as laundry, supplies, janitorial service, and other miscellaneous expenses

Indirect costs can be calculated by three commonly used methods:

- Equally used methods

- Indirect proportion to revenue generated by the service

- Indirect proportion to the direct cost of each service

To determine the *direct* and *indirect* costs, and before fees are set for each year, it is necessary for a practice to perform a direct cost analysis by revenue center. See Exhibit 2-1, *Cost Analysis by Service Worksheet* for an example of this review.

While it is not entirely necessary to analyze direct costs, this exercise will give you a more comprehensive view of the costs of delivering a specific service. Such costs should be allocated fairly and there should never be a "gouging" of allocation in order for one department or revenue center to look better than another. Many times this occurs if a bias exists toward a certain revenue center.

Exhibit 2-1 illustrates a simple worksheet to calculate the direct and indirect costs and actual profit by division generated for each revenue center. The contribution margin of the revenue center is calculated initially by subtracting the direct costs from the revenues. Then the indirect cost is applied to this amount with the difference being the division profit. Certain assumptions must be made based upon life expectancy of assets for purposes of depreciation, and cost per test for supplies, and an allocation of an employee's time (which may not be 100 percent) in the specific revenue center.

Cost Analysis By Service Worksheet

Exhibit 2-1

REVENUE/COST ANALYSIS FOR _____

Revenues $_____

Direct Cost

    Salary/Benefits [1] $_____

    Cost of Supplies $_____

    Supplies [2] $_____

    Equipment Depreciation [3] $_____

    Maintenance & Repairs $_____

    Total Direct Costs $_____

    Contribution Margin $_____

Indirect Costs

    Building Lease [4] $_____

    Utilities $_____

    Miscellaneous [5] $_____

    Total Direct Costs $_____

    Division Profit $_____

[1] Based on 80% of one employee's time.

[2] Based on $_____ per test.

[3] Based on _____ year life expectancy.

[4] Costs in this category are based on the proportion of square footage occupied by the equipment, if applicable.

[5] Janitorial, laundry, maintenance, property tax.

Cost Analysis by Item

Another viable way to analyze costs and gross margins of a practice is to use the *Costs Analysis by Item Worksheet*, Exhibit 2-2. The goal of this analysis is to determine the profit center's margin on a single service or item. The example illustrated in Exhibit 2-2 shows a current fee charge for a Gynecological exam, describing specific cost of supplies and other related direct costs for completing that exam. The net profit total, therefore, does not consider the cost of labor and other overhead items. Perform this quick exercise before setting fees for injections or certain service procedures.

Cost Analysis By Item Worksheet

Exhibit 2-2

Service	Current Fee	Cost of Supplies Needed		Net Profit
Gyn Exam	$55.00	Disposable Speculum	$1.20	$52.22
		Paper Gown	.65	
		Urine Cup	.25	
		K-Y Jelly	.03	
		Disposable Glove	.05	
		Drape Sheet	.25	
		Table Paper	.02	
			$2.45	
1.2 M.U. Bi-Cillin Inj.	$10.00	$5.50		$4.50

Cost Analysis per Patient

Another feasible method for measuring performance within the practice is calculating the cost per patient. Compute by using the following formula:

$$\underline{\textit{Total Expenses Less Occupancy Expenses, Physician and Staff Salaries and Benefits}}$$
$$\textit{Total Patients Seen}$$

Here is an example of this calculation, assuming the subsequent operating results:

- Gross charges, $450,000
- Collections, $379,000
- Expenses excluded from the calculation, $134,000
- Net expenses, $86,000 (These represent the total expenses to be considered in the cost per patient analysis, net of occupancy costs, physician and staff salaries and benefits.)

Assume also there are 6,500 patients seen per year. A simple computation of the cost per patient is:

$$\frac{\$86,000}{\$6,500} \quad = \quad \$13.23 \textit{ Cost Per Patient}$$

The reason occupancy expenses and physician and staff salaries and benefits are not a part of this calculation is to consider a cost per patient factor outside of the direct cost of personnel and renting office space. Occupancy expenses, and physician and staff salaries are not considered because they do not change with patient numbers (patients seen). In other words, establish a break even amount that encompasses all expenses prior to consideration of salaries, benefits and rent expense. Knowing this figure (the cost of care only) will enable the practice administrator and physician(s) to more accurately determine what they can afford to pay in salaries and rent expense in order to derive an acceptable gross margin for the practice.

Customized Cost Procedures Analysis

In a constantly changing reimbursement environment, relevant and timely information is essential for making informed decisions for the practice. The practice administrator and physician(s) must know the ten procedures that have the greatest profit margins in the practice. Similarly, it is important to know the ten procedures that have the smallest profit margins.

To help physicians attain this data, computerized procedure analysis systems have been developed. Normally, cost procedure analysis is a combination of a computer software analysis combined with professional consultative evaluations. Such customized evaluations can reveal extensive and pertinent information specific to the practice.

Current principles of cost accounting, such as standard costing and contribution margin analysis, are applied to the procedure mix. Because of the information generated by the analysis, decisions can be made that affect various situations. These considerations may range from managed care contracting to changing reimbursement strategies. Potentially, a cost procedure analysis enables the practice to increase net collections, adjust fee levels, track profitability, discover coding anomalies, forecast the impact of capitation, and obtain valuable information for assessment of the operations of the practice.

In most practices, a customized cost procedures analysis is beyond the practice administrator's responsibilities. Therefore, such services should be outsourced to a consulting firm with capabilities of completing the report. See Exhibit 2-3 as an example of the outcome of a Cost Procedure Analysis for a specific CPT code.

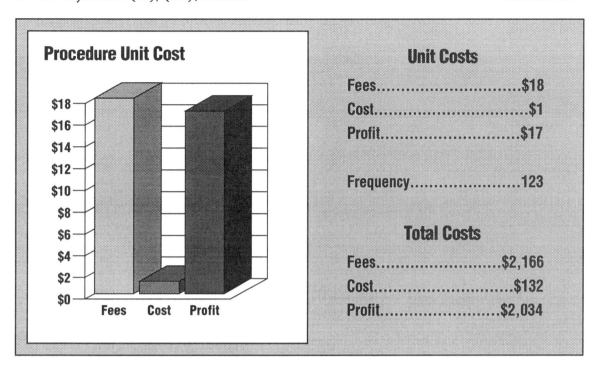

Procedure Unit Cost	Unit Costs	
	Fees	$18
	Cost	$1
	Profit	$17
	Frequency	123
	Total Costs	
	Fees	$2,166
	Cost	$132
	Profit	$2,034

The Summary Report

With today's advanced technology, software systems can generate volumes of data. Sometimes, the reports are too cumbersome for a busy physician or group of physicians to absorb. Instead of presenting comprehensive reports, the practice administrator can create a simple, one-page summary report for the physician(s) or other owners of the practice. This will provide the physician(s) with a "quick read" report, enabling them to keep a finger on the pulse of the practice. This review can be accomplished in a short period of time, perhaps 30 minutes or less.

To generate a summary report, you need a productivity analysis and the monthly financial statements. It is important that this information be completed as soon after the end of the month as possible. If you use an outside firm, such as a CPA, to complete the financial statements, you will need to provide them the information as soon as possible after month end. Arrangements should be made, prior to agreeing to give them the work, for the return of the completed financial statements no later than from the fifth to the seventh working days of each month. Generally, this timetable will facilitate your having the final summary report by the tenth calendar day of the month. The timeliness of receiving the financial statements and completing the summary report is requisite for you to react to certain situations that occurred in the previous month.

Refer to the following two reports that summarize key data within the practice; Exhibit 2-4, *Tracking Practice Growth and Profitability* and Exhibit 2-5, *Monthly Statistic Report*. Again, having a concisely summarized, two-page report provides the physician(s) or other owners of the practice with a quick, yet informative, analysis of the results of the practice operations.

	Goal	Current Month	Previous Month	YTD
Billings				
Collections				
Adjustments				
Collections Percentage (Fee-for-service cash collections ÷ Gross fee-for-service charges)				
Total Accounts Receivable				
Accounts Receivable Ratio (Total Accounts Receivable ÷ Average monthly billings)				
New Patients				
Total Patient Visits				
Expense Ratio (Total non-physician expense ÷ Total gross charges)				
Profit <Loss> (Collections minus expenses)				
Net Income Percentage (Total net income ÷ collections)				

In the first report (Exhibit 2-4), note that a "Goal" column has been placed to the left of the Current Month, Previous Month, and Year-to-Date (YTD) results. It is important to reflect this "Goal" or perhaps better stated, "Budgeted Total," in the summary report. In most cases, this column should be used as a measurement of the operating results for the current month. While it is good to know historical information as a comparison (such as the Previous Month), it is more significant to compare the current month operations against the budget or goal amounts.

Monthly Statistics Report   Exhibit 2-5

Month: _____

Total Charges: _____

Adjustments: _____

Net Charges: _____

Total Receipts: _____

Adjustments: _____

Net Receipts: _____

Total Patients Seen: _____

Daily Average: _____

Collection Ratio: _____

Accounts Receivable: _____

Average Per Patient Charge: _____

Average Per Patient Cost: _____

Total Monthly Expense: _____

Net Income: _____

The *Monthly Statistics Report* provides a summary of key practice data primarily involving total production, cash collected, and patients seen. The total monthly expense and net income of the practice for the month is also summarized at the end of the report.

These two summary reports serve as very useful management tools that probably will be used more by the physician(s) than other report they receive. In most cases, these two summary reports will become the key reporting mechanisms in lieu of a detailed review of the financial statements. While financial statements may be reviewed more on a quarterly, semi-annual, or annual basis, the summary reports will be helpful for monthly reviews.

CHAPTER 3

Controlling Overhead

Throughout this book, we have addressed the need to control expenses within the medical practice. This is more necessary now than at any other time in history, as managed care becomes a larger part of the revenue stream. Controlling expenses is mandatory as capitation rises to prominence as a means of payment to physicians. Further, as the government becomes more involved as a payor, and reimbursements scrutinized, if not eliminated, controlling overhead is ever more critical.

Medical practice overhead is directly related to the flow of patients, collections, and general structure of the practice. The fee schedule also has an influence on overhead. Standards for overhead are set by the physician(s). For example, there are "textbook" recommendations for staff size based on specialty, services rendered, etc. Yet the physician(s) may elect to have a larger staff than recommended. If the decision is made to employ a larger staff, there must also be acceptance of a higher expense ratio (assuming they are the owners of the practice). A practice administrator should assume the responsibility of objectively *informing* the physician(s) of recommended staffing levels and suggest alternatives. There may be other ways that expenses can be controlled or reduced that are not as onerous as eliminating employees. The role of a practice administrator is to determine opportunities for reducing overhead and to present them to management.

Expense-to-earnings ratio have consistently risen over the last several years. Recent articles and statistical data bank publications present "acceptable" overhead percentages. While noteworthy, the overhead of a medical practice should be that percentage of total revenues that allow the practice to operate efficiently yet produces an acceptable profit margin. This varies depending upon the geographical region, the physicians' background, years in practice, etc., and the willingness for the physician(s) to share some of their income with key employees. By paying higher salaries to employees or having more staff than is absolutely necessary, the practice's income is reduced. This affects the amount normally distributed to the physicians as a part of their total compensation. The final decision is with the owner(s)/physician(s).

High Overhead

What one person regards as high overhead may not seem out of line by another. However, generally high overhead percentages suggest one, if not all, of the following characteristics:

- Low patient volume; outdated and inequitable fee schedules.

- Inefficient administrative management and oversight resulting in excess expense.

- Over staffing; inefficient staffing (i.e., scheduling that does not lend itself to optimum levels of productivity).

- Poorly negotiated managed care contracts resulting in low reimbursement.
- Lack of discipline to manage expenses based upon goals or budgets.
- Lack of strategic planning and coordination of expense controls.

Low Overhead

Conversely, some practices have percentages of overhead that are too low. While this is normally seen to be a "positive" indication in terms of the practice's operations, it may actually indicate an underlying problem. An issue may eventually surface that results in less than acceptable performance in the future. Characteristics of low overhead percentages are:

- Inequitably high fees.
- Lack of proper patient management (e.g., skimping in the area of patient care).
- Failure to deliver high-quality medical care.
- Under staffing or low salary and low benefit standards.

These cost-saving initiatives can have a negative effect over time. Inequitably high fees in today's health care market will eventually be corrected either through a managed care scenario or through competition (i.e., loss of patients to another provider). Skimping in patient care increases the risk of malpractice liability claims. Under staffing or low salary and benefit standards promote constant turnover; and optimum productivity and efficiency among staff members is not reached. Ultimately, this limits the productivity of the physician(s).

Overhead Control Suggestions

In the operation and administration of a medical practice, there are many exercises to control overhead. Primarily, a practice must be run like any other business. This means making logical, well-thought decisions based on sufficient analyses. Many medical practices are run like traditional "mom and pop" businesses, and "difficult" decisions are avoided. While this may have worked in the past, there are new pressures on physicians to protect their level of income.

Following is a comprehensive list of overhead control suggestions. They are neither all-inclusive nor totally applicable to every practice. However, most are useful and, if adopted, will generate considerable savings over a year's time.

1. *Use a postage meter and scale.*
   Reduce mailing overhead at least 10–20 percent by using a postage meter and scale. When only stamps are used, there is a tendency for them to be misplaced or used for personal reasons. Less postage is wasted when an electronic scale is used.

2. *Use bulk mailing services when possible.*
   Consider using bulk mail when conducting a marketing campaign or handling other high volume mailings. Use the lowest rates applicable for mailing billing statements, such as pre-sorted first class postage. Ask at your local post office about any services available to lower the effective postage rate. Compare overnight shipping vendors; knowing what services and rates are available helps to control cost. Limit the use of overnight shipping as much as possible. Use a two- or three-day carrier service at a much cheaper rate.

3. *Type progress notes on self-stick paper and post into the chart.*
   This time saving measure reduces paper handling and duplication of labor.

4. *When possible, use the telephone instead of written correspondence.*
   Lengthy long distance telephone usage is expensive and must be used with discretion. However, written correspondence takes much more time and effort and requires time spent by both the physician and the employee who generates the letter.

5. *Use a high school student for filing and other simple, clerical duties.*
   Hire an individual who is 17 years of age or older to work for minimum wage or a rate slightly above.

6. *Purchase or lease the practice's telephone system.*
   Buying or leasing equipment costs no more than entering a straight rental agreement. After the system is paid for, expenses will be reduced.

7. *Use a discount long distance telephone carrier.*
   Investigate and analyze long distance service options. The competitive marketplace provides excellent opportunities for savings.

8. *Prepare a patient information brochure.*
   Prepare a patient information brochure to answer questions about the practice and to serve as a marketing and promotion tool. This information will reduce the volume of incoming calls and improve patient relations.

9. *Be aware of energy savings.*
   Save money over the course of a year by turning thermostats up in the summer and down in the winter. Turn off lights and equipment when not in use.

10. *Avoid over use of utilities.*
    Make a conscious effort to conserve water, gas, and other utilities.

11. *Check for under utilization of diagnostic equipment.*
    Equipment of any nature is expensive to own and maintain. If such equipment is seldom used or not needed, it should be eliminated. Consider sharing equipment with other practices, if appropriate.

12. *Consider bank accounts that are interest bearing.*
    Most operating accounts pay interest on the balance. This offsets service charges that may apply.

13. *Manage cash efficiently.*
    Besides having an ongoing operating bank account, each practice should maintain a separate investment account that earns a higher rate of interest. Transfer excess funds to the investment account to maximize the return. Be sure these funds can be liquidated without incurring penalties. Inevitably, the cash will be needed for operating expenses or disbursement to the physicians. Do not pay bills before the due date.

14. *Cross train office and clinical staff for coverage during time off.*
    Cross training of employees is a fundamental cost savings measure. Eliminate the need to hire temporary replacement personnel during absences due to vacation and illness by assigning responsibilities to trained staff members.

15. *Pay employees on an hourly basis instead of salary.*
Consider paying nonexempt employees on an hourly basis rather than by salary. Establish a system to control unsubstantiated requests for overtime pay.

16. *Use a time clock to record employees work hours.*
Avert overestimation of time worked by having employees "clock in" and "clock out" at the beginning and end of the work day. Be certain that time worked is not cushioned by employees who choose to arrive early, clock in and drink coffee for the first few minutes. Similarly, discourage those who delay leaving at the end of the day to increase their pay. It may be necessary to monitor the actual clocking in and out of employees.

17. *Use merit and performance guidelines for staff salary increases.*
Complete an annual review for each employee. Use standard forms for documentation of performance. Never sign a performance review form that is based on undocumented and unsubstantiated opinion. Keep good notes and fully document key discussions that occur during the appraisal review.

18. *Keep wage increases in line with inflation rates.*
This is not to say that a raise that exceeds the rate of inflation should not be given to a deserving employee. An employee who performs in such a way to justify a higher raise should receive one, if agreeable to all in management. Annual raises should be given based on a percentage. An employee develops expectations, from one year to the next, based upon the previous year's percentage increases. Once a particularly large increase is received, expectations are in place for subsequent years. When giving a large increase, explain the exceptional reason or circumstance; illustrate why it is higher than previous or possibly subsequent years. Most employees will understand these conditions if properly apprised at the time.

19. *Provide basic employee fringe benefits but do not overdo when unnecessary.*
Some employees are in the work force primarily to receive employee benefits, particularly health insurance. On the other hand, some employees have less need for fringe benefits provided by their employer. If an individual is able to participate in a plan offered through his/her spouse's employer, there may be no interest in dual coverage. It is very difficult for a small medical practice to provide fringe benefits to employees at a reasonable cost. Therefore, rather than providing extensive benefits, consider paying higher base salaries. This allows employees to purchase their own benefits, if needed, by offsetting the expense. Otherwise, they have additional discretionary income to spend.

Employee benefit plans are a major expense for any business, including a medical practice. Before committing to providing a benefit, use extreme caution; review the plan carefully. It is not necessarily a requirement of a new practice to provide benefits, however, once a benefit program begins, employees have a perception of "entitlement." Therefore, consider delaying this expense until the practice is well established.

20. *Evaluate each employee's qualifications and determine them to be commensurate with the job.*
Overqualified employees are likely to be costly to the practice. In hiring and in managing, closely align qualifications with job descriptions. An employee who is over qualified either expects a higher level of income or eventually leaves to find a job that better suits him/her. Turnover is a costly hidden expense within the practice. Hiring, training, and developing an individual to replace a previous employee requires a significant investment.

21. *Charge for consultation work.*

Generate income by billing for the physicians' professional services that occur outside the realm of medical practice. Examples of such services are charging insurance companies for time to prepare medical reports; charging attorneys or other entities for depositions and for testifying as an expert witness in a trial; earning honoraria for speaking engagements and presentations.

22. *Use an order list for supplies rather than ordering randomly.*

Prevent unnecessary ordering of supplies by using a form/list. A suitable supply form has the following features: (1) a preprinted list of supplies frequently ordered; (2) a column with spaces for current inventory; (3) a column to requisition items needed; (4) space for ordering additional items; (5) and an approval line to be signed by the practice administrator. As an additional cost savings measure, discourage employees from using office supplies for personal use.

23. *Use competitive bid lists to compare vendors; obtain references for larger vendors.*

Compare price lists of various vendors. Competition keeps prices low. Vary the use of vendors for the same supply items to maintain a level of competition and pricing control.

24. *Set up a supply/reorder system based upon need level only.*

Requisition supplies using a current inventory listing on the requisition form. (See item Number 22.) This eliminates over ordering or ordering when unnecessary just because "new" supplies are wanted.

25. *Review insurance policies to see if lower premiums are available.*

Using brokers who represent several companies, review policy options at least annually. Do not sacrifice adequate coverage for lower premiums. Be certain to maintain adequate insurance protection, particularly for liability purposes. Malpractice liability insurance rates vary significantly by state and by specialty. Some companies offer discounts through associations or other organizations. Consider various options and watch for opportunities to save in this very expensive, yet needed, area.

26. *Keep up-to-date job descriptions.*

Update job descriptions as job assignments change or as new roles emerge. Be sure that the job description and the employee's qualifications are good matches, and see that higher paid workers are not doing lower paid work.

27. *Hire the level of expertise, training, and experience needed to do the particular job.*

Do not hire an RN if a qualified LPN or Medical Assistant can perform the task equally well at a lower salary.

28 *Avoid overtime pay unless overtime is actually worked.*

Require all overtime work to be preapproved by the practice administrator. This preapproval process deters employees from claiming overtime for quarter and half hour segments of time. It also discourages mismanagement of one's time, particularly when clocking in and out.

29. *Try to motivate employees to avert turnover.*

Motivate employees through fair and equitable supervision and treatment. Institute training programs and upgrade qualifications and work responsibilities whenever appropriate. Use a very hands-on management approach to growing and developing employees talents. Turnover is often caused by employees not feeling trained to do their job well.

30. *Employ an independent payroll service to reduce manager, bookkeeping, or accounting time.*

Consider saving money and increasing efficiency by using an outside payroll service. Using an outside service also helps to preserve confidentiality of salaries.

31. *Utilize a consultant/accountant for assistance in review and interpretation of financial statements.*

Use an outside consultant or CPA to prepare financial statements. Preparation of these reports requires special training or close supervision by a degreed professional accountant. Financial statements provided at least quarterly, if not monthly, are indispensable management tools. These statements should include budgeted totals as comparative data with actual performing operating results. Financial statements prepared using generally accepted accounting principles assure an accurate depiction of the operating results and simplify the preparation of year-end tax returns for both the practice and the physicians.

32. *Manage office space efficiently.*

Consider subletting excess office space, if appropriate, or negotiating a rental reduction. Keep occupancy costs as low as possible; these savings directly affect net profits. Persuade the landlord to underwrite some of the ongoing cost of operations, e.g., sharing of utilities, and paying for tenant improvements. In exchange, consider signing a longer term lease. Be sure this fits with the practice's strategic plan.

33. *Negotiate for a one-year requirement of supplies to secure a lower price.*

Take advantage of lower pricing through higher volume purchasing. Consider joining buying consortiums or associations that have negotiated discounts with vendors.

34. *Plan all major purchases according to your annual operating budget.*

Delay buying non-budgeted capital items; purchase only after significant review and after agreement is reached among the owners of the practice.

35. *Purchase minor supplies (pens, pencils, paper clips) from discount houses, such as membership warehouses.*

Small office supply companies generally charge higher prices to cover delivery costs.

36. *Consider buying interesting books for the reception area instead of weekly/monthly magazines.*

Books cost less than magazines subscriptions that must be renewed. Generally, books lend less clutter to the waiting area.

37. *Consult your professional financial advisor before leasing equipment or making a significant purchase.*

While leasing is not always the way to acquire an item, often it makes the most sense. Leasing, which is nothing more than another way to finance a purchase, always includes an imputed interest factor. Weigh this factor against a straight purchase of the item. How will this affect your line of credit at your bank? What interest rate will be charged on the bank loan? Compare the total cost; the lease may be more expensive. A lease will not access a practice's line of credit and, therefore, will not reduce the amount available to borrow for other things. In some situations, this may justify a leasing decision rather than opting to purchase by borrowing the money on a line of credit.

38. *Negotiate collection agency fees and bank card rates.*
Agency fees and bank card rates are negotiable items that vary with volume. Do not assume that the rates quoted are the best available; many agencies discount rates, when asked. Obtain comparative information about rates attained by other practices before accepting quotes. Secure bids from several collection agencies for the assurance of receiving competitive pricing.

39. *Make sure that the hospitals are responsive to the physicians.*
Make sure that hospitals know the importance of helping the physician(s) in the management of his/her time, particularly while making rounds at the hospital. This helps physicians optimize their productivity in the practice. Less time spent at the hospital means more time available at the office for seeing patients and generating revenue.

40. *Review ratios and trends for revenues and expenses at least quarterly.*
Compare ratios and trends against the prior year's actual results and current year's budget. This exercise is essential to controlling overhead and managing the practice. All owners, including the physicians of the practice, should complete this activity. The practice administrator should submit concise summary reports to the physicians monthly. *(See Chapter 6.)*

41. *Work with the outside consultant to prepare and update annually a strategic plan for the practice.*
An up-to-date strategic plan helps the owners/physicians ascertain the current position of the practice and hopefully where it is going in the future.

Checklist for a Profitable Practice

A clear-cut message emerges as we discuss ways to control overhead and as we consider ways to identify operational efficiencies. That message is, *a profitable, successful medical practice no longer happens by chance.* It requires planning, analysis, forethought and a defined direction. Summarized below is a checklist for operating a profitable practice. Answer each question. If your answer affirms an efficient operation, be assured of success.

- ✔ Does your financial recordkeeping give complete information about your practice?

- ✔ Do you have a method of reviewing expenses to determine ways to reduce costs?

- ✔ Do you understand the basics of financial statements, what they mean and what is important in them?

- ✔ Does your current information system help you plan and make decisions?

- ✔ Is your computer software up-to-date and manageable?

- ✔ Does your independent consultant or accountant help you review financial statements?

- ✔ Does your independent consultant or accountant help you analyze trends?

- ✔ Does your practice administrator attempt to learn the meaning of the financial statements and the trends that can be understood from their review?

- ✔ Do the physicians acquaint themselves with the operations of the practice and the financial results?

- ✔ Do you have good communication with your office personnel?

- ✔ Is your office staff cross trained?

✔ Is there any one employee who is truly indispensable?

✔ Is your current staff meeting the standards that have been set?

✔ Do you have a policy of regular performance evaluations of personnel?

✔ Are all members of your staff held accountable for their actions and performance?

✔ Do you have specific ways to motivate and encourage employees to perform well?

✔ Are incentives provided to help motivate your personnel?

✔ Do you set the standards for work with a high work ethic?

✔ Do you allow employees to enjoy their jobs while being productive?

✔ Do you promote growth and development of your employees?

✔ Do you allow employees to speak their mind and feel comfortable in recommending improvements to the practice?

✔ Are you satisfied with how your employees are working together?

✔ Do you have an organized policy on employee benefits and compensation?

✔ Are the physicians within the practice considerate of the employees?

✔ Are the physicians within the practice considerate of each other?

✔ Does an overriding theme exist within the practice, that serving the patient is the number one priority?

✔ Do your patients clearly understand your billing policies and insurance processing?

✔ Do your patients respect the physicians and staff because of the way they are treated?

✔ Do your patients believe that the physicians within the practice are only interested in making more money?

✔ In general, does your practice demonstrate excellent patient/staff relations?

✔ Is your staff trained thoroughly on your billing policy and do they follow it closely?

✔ Are you cognizant of fully documenting all procedures performed in order to bill the maximum?

✔ Are you attempting to only perform procedures necessary, or do you over utilize at times?

✔ Are you satisfied with all aspects of your medical record system?

✔ Is your staff managing third party billing efficiently?

✔ Are you satisfied with your direction regarding managed care contracting?

✔ Are you satisfied with your current payor mix?

✔ Is there opportunity to increase your fees through a basic fee analysis, particularly in the area of indemnity insurers?

✔ Does your appointment scheduling work satisfactorily?

✔ Does your receptionist maximize the scheduling process?

✔ Does the receptionist follow up on "no shows?"

✔ Does your appointment scheduling process need to be automated?

✔ Is the patient volume as you like it?

✔ Is the marketing of your practice what it should be?

✔ Does the community know of your practice? What can be done to better acquaint them with it?

✔ Are the hospitals in which you practice assisting in the development of your practice?

✔ Is the waiting time for patients a problem?

✔ Do you get regular feedback and appraisals from staff about your practice?

✔ Does the staff respond to the physicians request to maximize their operational efficiency toward patients?

✔ Are collections where they should be?

✔ Do you write off to bad debts a large amount of accounts receivable every month?

✔ How strong is your balance sheet? Do you have to borrow money regularly to meet working capital needs?

✔ Do you use an outside collection agency to follow up on and collect unpaid account balances?

✔ Do you want to continue to practice medicine privately (if this is a private practice) or do you consider it an option to sell the practice and become an employed physician?

✔ Are you in a call group with other physicians that complements the way you practice medicine?

✔ Do you have to "moonlight" at the hospital emergency room or another ancillary work in order to earn a total income that you expect to make as a physician?

✔ Are you actively involved with the hospital's medical staff?

✔ Are you actively involved with civic projects, memberships, public speaking engagements, etc., in the community where you live and work?

✔ Is your practice in compliance with the regulatory requirements of Occupational Safety & Health Administration (OSHA) and the Americans with Disabilities Act (ADA)?

✔ Do you have a plan of operation that dedicates investment of retained earnings to office refurbishment and upgrades to assure an up-to-date image?

✔ Do you have a Personnel Policy and Procedures Manual, and is it kept up-to-date?

✔ Have you taken advantage of all possible reimbursement enhancement opportunities (e.g., rural health clinic certification, fee schedule adjustments that coincide with ceilings for reimbursements set by indemnity insurers, etc.)?

✔ Do you have adequate cash controls in existence to insure that there is no embezzlement of practice funds?

✔ Do you have checks and balances in place to approve refunds to patients?

✔ Do you personally approve charity and professional courtesies write-offs?

✔ Do you require all checks to be signed with a dual signature or only a physician's?

✔ Can you improve reimbursement cash flow by filing claims electronically?

✔ Can you improve cash flow regarding secondary filings through more efficient paperwork processing?

✔ Do you know and understand the demographics of your practice?

✔ Do you believe your practice is slanted too much in the direction of one age group or payor mix than another?

✔ Are you using a financial planner to help you in developing your retirement program? Are you allowing a tax consultant to assist you in reducing the tax liability generated from your practice?

CHAPTER 4

Internal Control Systems

Cash Flow Management

Conservation and effective use of cash are essential to the operation of any medical practice. Unfortunately, often cash is not managed well due to the small number of employees and a general lack of appropriate controls. There is a greater potential for fraudulent activities in medical practices than in other businesses.

Cash flow management is critical with any small business. The medical practice particularly is faced with the need for better management more than ever before. As reimbursements are reduced, and the payors are better managing their cash disbursements, increased pressure is placed on the practice to maintain a constant flow of cash. Since most medical practices are privately owned and operated by the physicians, when cash flow becomes tight or negative, the physicians must supplement the shortfall. This is a source of frustration for the physician(s)/owner(s).

Strong controls must be in place to maximize collections and to maintain internal control over them. Neither component should be de-emphasized. However, in an effort to maximize collections, some internal controls may be sacrificed. Weigh these decisions in the balance of other time demands within the practice, knowing the personnel involved and level of trust.

Banking Relationships and Bank Accounts

Generally, each practice should establish and use two bank accounts.

- **Regular operating account**
  Maintain a cash balance operating account for regular disbursements of accounts payable and payroll. Keep only enough money in this account to avert usage charges, plus an additional cushion to cover incidental checks that are written throughout the month. When paying the monthly accounts payable, transfer just enough money from the money market account to the operating account to cover the dollar amount of the checks written In addition, this should be done for the payroll whether or not a separate account is maintained for it.

- **Money market account**
  Money market accounts have a higher yield than most interest bearing checking accounts, and deposits begin earning interest immediately. Use this account for excess cash flow. It should be liquid enough to allow movement of funds to the operating account and ultimately for disbursement to the physicians/owners.

- **Payroll account**

  Larger practices that have several employees (i.e., 10 or more) should establish a separate payroll account. This can be a "zero" balance account in which only enough money is transferred to offset the payroll for each pay period. If direct deposit is made for payroll, consider arranging with your bank for an automatic transfer of the total balance. If a separate payroll account is not used, emphasis should be placed on maintaining confidentiality. Limit the number of authorized signers and individuals who have access to the account, including the reconciliation of it.

Managing Incoming Cash

Following are some points to remember in the operation and management of incoming cash:

- Deposit collections (checks and cash payments) daily, unless the amounts are so small it does not warrant the effort. Prepare a deposit slip every day and show a total for that day. If you skip a day making a deposit, make two deposits the next day. This provides a verification that all funds received on a day was deposited in total.

- Copy insurance and attach explanation of benefits.

- Copy patient checks and attach to *Daily Collections Summary Worksheet (see Exhibit 4-3)*.

- Record each receivable separately on the deposit slip. While this may take more time, it leaves a good audit trail and serves as proper documentation for posting the receivable. Often, this can be posted using a computer software program and the subsequent report used as a summary backup sheet to the deposit slip.

- Enter the check number for bulk checks. This allows for matching a particular check to the Explanation of Monthly Benefits statement that came with it. It also provides a tracking of payment, if needed.

- Manage cash flow daily. A basic summary sheet to track cash flow can be easily completed. Summarize as follows: **beginning balance plus (+) deposits current day less (-) disbursements current day equal (=) ending balance.** Reconcile to the bank statement and financial statement book balance each month to be certain an accurate daily "cash flash" exists.

- Look at trends to anticipate cash inflow and outflow. Most practices have fairly consistent disbursements, and over time and within a particular period during the year, incoming cash is predictable.

- Pay accounts payable on a timely basis, but never early unless discounts are such that it makes sense to do so and the cash is available.

- Secure a working capital line of credit with your bank. This provides a fallback when working capital is short and borrowing is necessary.

In summary, cash management is a daily occurrence. The practice administrator assumes this responsibility and reports to the physician(s)/owners. If the job is being done regularly, there are no surprises or embarrassing times when cash is short. An exception occurs if the practice is simply not producing enough cash to justify its expenses. This will be detected early with good forward cash management.

Petty Cash Policy

Briefly, let's look at a petty cash policy. A petty cash fund provides a small source of cash to pay amounts that are impractical to pay by check. Here are some recommended controls for maintaining a petty cash fund.

Determine the amount to be placed in the petty cash fund. A small amount works well, normally $50.00 or less, allowing for reimbursement at relatively short intervals. Purchase a lockable box and a supply of "Received of Petty Cash" forms from an office supply store. Consider these rules and policies:

- Responsibility for the fund should be vested to the practice administrator or managing physician of the practice.

- Numbered and signed "Received of Petty Cash" forms should be obtained and all documentation for disbursements should be written in ink.

- Whenever petty cash is disbursed, the amount, date, and purpose should be entered and a "Received of Petty Cash" form kept with the remaining cash. Include a receipt for each amount paid from the fund to document the expenditure.

- The actual cash plus payments (the value of the slips and receipts) should always equal the predetermined amount of the petty cash fund.

- Maintain a log of petty cash disbursements indicating receipt number, date, and the item purchased. Start with the beginning balance and subtract disbursements to maintain a running balance of the cash receipts. See Exhibit 4-1, *Petty Cash Reconciliation Form* for an example.

			(B)	**(C)**
Disbursements	**Date Starting:** _____ **Date Ending:** _____			
	(A) Starting Balance $ _____			
No.	**Date**	**Item Purchased**	**Amount**	**Balance**
		Total		

Total Transactions: (A)   –   (B)   =   (C)

                    $ _____ $ _____ $ _____

Request for Reimbursement: $ _____

Submitted By: _____   Date: _____

- The practice administrator or appointed physician should approve all disbursements from petty cash.

- The petty cash fund should be counted and balanced (if feasible, by an employee other than the petty cash custodian) at the time of reimbursement of the fund.

- Personal checks of the employees should not be cashed in the petty cash fund.

- Advances to employees should never be paid out of the petty cash fund nor should IOUs be placed in the petty cash fund.

- At regular intervals, a check to "Petty Cash" should be written for the sum of "Received of Petty Cash" forms and receipts. Staple this documentation to the Petty Cash Reconciliation Form for verification.

Internal Checks and Balances for Cash Management

Within a typical medical practice, routine transactions involving cash receipts include:

- Cash and checks received through the mail (e.g., from patients, insurance companies, managed care companies, administrators from insurance plans, Medicare and Medicaid payments, and miscellaneous proceeds).

- Over-the-counter receipts from patients paid at the time of visit.

- Over-the-counter collections on account.

- Monies credited to the practice's bank account for payments received from bank cards and other charge cards, including Visa, MasterCard, American Express, etc.

The system of internal checks and balances assures that both innocent errors and deliberate fraud do not occur. The key is to separate handling of cash from the accounting records. One employee receives the cash; another posts it to the books; and another deposits it at the bank.

There are certain key balancing totals that may be easily and quickly reviewed daily by the practice administrator (and occasionally by the physician). These totals will verify that the day's collections are accurately recorded and safely (and fully) deposited in the practice's operating bank account.

An internal control system must be tailored to the individual practice. While many "textbook" controls sound good (and are in theory), each practice must translate them into a practical, realistic, and economically prudent approach to duties, assignments, and responsibilities. Consult an outside accountant or CPA who is familiar with your practice for advice in establishing appropriate internal controls. This unbiased, objective approach from an outsider lends credibility to this process.

Both the employer and employee benefit from strict internal controls. Individuals work without suspicion of fraud. Simultaneously, good internal controls provide early detection of loss due to errors. Most of the lapses that occur are not due to intentional fraudulent activities; they are due to innocent mistakes or carelessness. Internal controls avert these errors and potential intentional fraudulent activities.

When a practice establishes internal control guidelines, exceptions should rarely, if ever, occur. Guidelines do no good unless they are followed daily. General recommendations for controlling cash and maintaining good internal controls include the following:

- The employee opening the mail records all payments received through the mail in a *Mail Receipts Journal* (see Exhibit 4-2) before transferring them to the employee making the deposit. The Journal includes a section for itemizing payments not directly related to patient accounts (e.g., fees for depositions or copies of records to insurance companies, etc.). Periodically, the practice administrator reconciles these records with the actual deposit slip.

- Cash paid to physicians for services not connected with the practice should not be included in the practice deposits. These include such things as honoraria, rental income, interest income, or any other non-physician professionally generated fees. Give these monies directly to the physician. Maintain a log to track these payments as they are received. Any income not related to patients' fees (e.g., copies of medical records) deposited into the practice operating account, must be posted to the daily journal to reconcile charges and receipts and to prevent overstatement of the collection rate at month- and year-end.

- Procedures for handling cash should be clearly defined and responsibilities specifically assigned, not left to the first employee who can get to it each day. Rotate these job functions on a periodic basis.

- The function of cash collections and cash disbursements should each be assigned to an employee (i.e., the same employee should not handle collections [A/R] and disbursements [A/P]).

- The handling of cash should be totally separate from records maintenance. Thus the employee opening the mail, counting the receipts, and making the daily deposit, should **not** be posting those receipts against the accounts receivable.

- All bank account reconciliations should be completed by someone who does not handle the cash or maintain the accounting records. Preferably, an outside accountant or CPA who regularly prepares financial statements for the practice will complete these reconciliations. All staff members, including the practice administrator, should be accountable to someone. This establishes accountability even if it is to an outside consultant.

- All employees involved in the handling of cash for the accounting records must take periodic vacations. During this absence, another employee should handle those functions. Periodic, unannounced job shifting should occur to expose or possibly prevent collusion.

- All employees handling cash or accounting records should be bonded. The need for this varies with the size of the practice and individual situation. Consider purchasing office overhead (employee dishonesty) insurance, if economically feasible.

- Statements mailed to patients or other payors must be prepared and mailed by an employee other than the cashier. Include instructions on the statement about whom to call in case of questions. If the person who makes the deposits also does the billing, an opportunity is provided to cover up, mispost, and reallocate funds.

- Cash payments received on the day of treatment should be charged to the accounts receivable ledger and simultaneously credited. Otherwise, dishonest employees may use opportunities such as this for theft. The actual payments that day, some of which may be in cash, are more easily stolen and covered up (recordkeeping-wise) if controls are not in place.

- At the end of each day, patient encounter forms and receipts should be collected and reconciled with the over-the-counter cash receipts.

  - For over-the-counter cash payments on account (not at the time of service), a prenumbered duplicate receipt should be filled out with one copy given to the patient.

  - Encounter forms should be prenumbered and prepared for each patient expected on a given day. "Walk-ins" should be issued an encounter form in the proper numerical sequence to those issued for scheduled patients.

  - At the end of each day, all encounter forms should be collected and placed in numerical sequence. Include forms issued for "no shows." Account for all forms. Do not destroy unused encounter forms.

  - Over-the-counter collections (cash, check, and credit card payments) should be totaled separately from mailed receipts. Attach the calculator tape to the batch of encounter forms and receipts and give them to the practice administrator. The total payment shown on the encounter forms and receipts should equal the total of the over-the-counter receipts for that day.

– Accounts receivable posting may be done at the time of service or at the end of the day when all encounter forms and receipts are collected.

Payments received through the mail should be posted in a *Mail Receipts Journal*. An example of a completed Journal, is illustrated in Exhibit 4-2.

Mail Receipts Journal   Exhibit 4-2

Mail Receipts Journal				*Receipts of January 20, 19xx*
Check/Reference Number, etc.	**Source**	**Sender**	**City/State**	**Amount**
560060	Check	Cigna Health Plan/HMO	Atlanta, GA	$5,630.00
19060	Check	Group Resources, Inc./TPA	Norcross, GA	460.00
220460	Check	Great-West Insurance Co.	Atlanta, GA	860.00
335	Check	Kay Antly	Alpharetta, GA	100.00
1.00890	Check	U.S. Govt./Medicare	Atlanta, GA	1,550.00
Other Income 220471	Check	Blue Cross/GA – deposition fee	Atlanta, GA	500.00
Total				$9,100.00

Prepared By:_____J.M.R._____   Date:_____1/20/xx_____

Explanation of Headings:

Check/Reference Number: Patient or other payor's prenumbered check or other voucher number on payment advice.

Source: Type of payment, such as cash, check, draft, bank credit, credit card. (Typically, these will be assigned a number in a computerized journal system.)

Sender: Name of patient and/or other payor, including insurance company, governmental institution, managed care administrator, etc. (Again, use assigned number system for a computerized journal.)

City/State and Amount: Self-explanatory.

Ideally, the *Mail Receipts Journal* is prepared by the employee responsible for opening the mail each day. This report may be formulated manually or by using a computer spread sheet. Provide three copies and distribute as follows:

- One copy to the employee who will prepare and make the bank deposits (envelopes and other remittance slips included).

- One copy to the accounting department for posting to the practice's financial records, including its accounts receivable ledger.

- One copy to the employee who prepares the journal.

Maintain these file copies for two years.

An example of a *Daily Collections Summary Worksheet* is illustrated in Exhibit 4-3. This is a simple form that shows relevant information about each payment received. The accounts receivable clerk records the cash received from the Mail Receipts Journal, plus the over-the-counter collections on this *Daily Collections Summary Worksheet*. This form may be incorporated into a computerized spreadsheet. Use the following checks and balances to review the collections and cash receipts process daily:

- The daily bank deposit must equal the *Daily Collections Summary Worksheet* total.

- The total credits to accounts receivable for each day should equal the net cash deposit at the bank and the total on the *Daily Collections Summary Worksheet*.

- Non-patient related collections (i.e., deposition fees, copies of records to insurance companies, etc.) should be included in this total as a separate line item on the *Daily Collections Summary Worksheet*.

- The total of the mail receipts should equal the daily deposit amount adjusted by the cash collected at the time of seeing a patient or other payments made on account by patients at the practice.

- A daily reconciliation of the accounts receivable total should be completed *(see Exhibit 4-4)*.

Daily Collections Summary Worksheet   Exhibit 4-3

Date: _____

Check No.	Description/ Patient Name	Physician	Cash	Check	Credit Card	Total	Payment Received

Daily Collections Summary Worksheet

Date: _____January 20, 19xx_____

Check No.	Description/ Patient Name	Physician	Cash	Check	Credit Card	Total	Payment Received
N/A	John Patrick	Russell	$30.00			$30.00	In Person
102	Mark Alan	Allums		$150.00		$150.00	In Person
N/A	American Express Payment	All doctors			$1,810.00	$1,810.00	In Person
560060	Cigna Health Plan/HMO	All doctors		$5,630.00		$5,630.00	Mail
19060	Group Resources, Inc./TPA for Kim Smith, patient	Underwood		$460.00		$460.00	Mail
220460	Great-West Insurance Co. for Jean Cagle, patient	Russell		$860.00		$860.00	Mail
335	Kay Antly	Allums		$100.00		$100.00	Mail
100890	U.S. Govt, Dept of HHS, Medicare Div. for Bob Taylor, patient	Underwood		$1,550.00		$1,550.00	Mail
220471	Blue Cross/GA – Deposition fee	Jordan		$500.00		$500.00	Mail
Total Days Receipts			**$30.00**	**$9,250.00**	**$1,810.00**	**$11,090.00**	
Credit Card Deposit						**$1,810.00**	
Net Cash Bank Deposit						**$11,090.00***	
Cash Received In Person						**<$1,990.00>**	
Net Cash Received by Mail						**$9,100.00****	

*Reconcile with daily bank deposit slip
**Reconcile with total on daily *Mail Receipts Journal (See Exhibit 4-2)*

Fraud and Dishonesty

Embezzlement is a problem that occurs often in a medical practice and poses a significant threat to a practice's resources. Watch for situations that increase the risk of misappropriation within the practice. Establish controls to guard against the potential for loss. Some ways funds are misappropriated are listed below.

Mail Receipts

Lapping — diverting practice funds and reporting them at some time after collection. Usually funds received from one account are credited against another one from which cash has previously been diverted.

Temporarily Using Practice Funds — "borrowing" without falsifying records. Cash is diverted for personal use with the intention of paying it back later. The payback may or may not occur. Chances are, if the employee thinks he/she has gotten away with it, he/she will justify or rationalize not replacing the money.

Bad Debt Charged Off Improperly — Charging off a patient's account balance and pocketing the cash from a payment. (All write-offs must have a supervisor's approval in writing before posting. The physician and/or outside consultant should initial the write-offs, as well.)

Excluding Miscellaneous Income — diverting monies by not reporting small amounts received (e.g., payment for deposition fees, fees for copies of records, etc.).

Over-the-Counter Sales

Fraud occurs when an employee fails to report (and keeps) all proceeds from cash received from patients who paid in person. ***Fraud also occurs when a smaller fee is posted rather than the true amount of the charge.***

What are the reasons for fraud? Often embezzlement or fraudulent activity is not committed because employees are inherently dishonest or have planned to do this from the beginning of their employment. Mostly, fraud results from an employee experiencing external economic pressures. Or an employee may perceive that he/she has not been dealt with fairly (i.e., has not received a raise due, etc.). In other cases, an employee is faced with a temptation he/she cannot withstand. These are the logical reasons why fraud occurs. For an explicit understanding of how the stage is set for fraudulent activities, consider the following:

- Internal controls are poor or nonexistent. For example:
  - controls are stated but not enforced; lapses are allowed to occur.
  - offenders go unpunished.
  - examples of high ethical conduct are not set.

- Individual employees have significant, personal financial pressures due to:
  - personal indebtedness.
  - lifestyle behavior (excessive drinking, gambling, drug use, etc.).
  - extravagant living standards.

- Employees believe they have been mistreated. For example,
  - low or no salary increases have been given.
  - benefits have been reduced (e.g., increase in health insurance premiums, etc.).

- Employees believe physicians are greedy and that they do not share profits with the employees.

- Employees hold the attitude that "they'll never miss it."

Deterring Embezzlement Activity

Following is a list of possible ways to reduce the risk of fraudulent activities and prevent embezzlement of practice funds.

1. Set up written control procedures and make sure employees follow them.

2. Avoid allowing one employee to have complete control over the entire sequence of cash transactions.

3. Limit access of cash to specified employees.

4. Make sure accounting records are kept by employees who do not handle receipts or cash disbursements.

5. If segregation of duties is impractical, make sure all work is periodically reviewed.

6. Have outside accountants perform periodic test checks and auditing reviews.

7. Regularly review contractual assignments, daily activity reports, and appointment calendars.

8. Periodically follow a random sampling of patients through the office from the charge ticket and the day sheet to the bank deposit.

9. Make sure that all bank accounts are balanced monthly.

10. Used prenumbered checks and superbills.

11. Keep records of all cash receipts and deposit them daily. Do not make payments out of undeposited receipts.

12. Compare cash receipts posted into your (coumputerized) system to the cash actually deposited in the bank.

13. Keep tight controls over petty cash. Make cash payments by check whenever possible.

14. Make sure the employee who signs checks is not the same employee who makes bank deposits and that the check signer has the opportunity to review supporting documentation (i.e., invoices).

15. Stamp checks "For Deposit Only" when they are received.

16. Require employees to take vacations. (Embezzlers are often caught when they are not around to cover their tracks.)

17. Keep an eye on employees who are having personal problems (for example, divorce, financial difficulty, etc.).

18. Provide adequate instructions to patients regarding the proper mailing of check remittances with instructions to make payable to the practice, not an individual or a physician.

19. Require employees to provide a written receipt to patients who make over-the-counter payment for services rendered on a different day. If a rubber stamp is used in the "pay to the order of" portion of the check, require that it be stamped in the presence of the patient who is paying. Ask patients to fill out the line on the check indicating for what the payment is being made. Consider posting these instructions at the front desk.

20. Consider purchasing bonding insurance for employees.

21. Follow up past due accounts promptly.

Finally, there are early warning signs to detect fraud if we just take the time to observe and "see the forest for the trees." Watch for these early warning signals:

1. The employee who never takes vacations.

2. The employee who insists on doing everything himself/herself.

3. The employee who is obviously living beyond his/her means.

4. The employee who expresses, "We do all the work, and they get all the money!"

5. Two employees with access to receipts who frequently arrange to make deposits together (i.e., the employee who opens the mail and the one who prepares the bank deposit).

6. The employee who is openly critical of the practice and in particular, its physicians/owners.

Summary

Internal controls and sound cash planning form the backbone of an efficiently operated medical practice. Physicians may deliver the highest quality health care services and generate substantial revenues. Whatever the production level, the funds must be collected, properly placed in the operating account, and then prudently managed to achieve *practice success!*

CHAPTER 5

Understanding Financial Statements

Income Statement and Balance Sheet

An *Income Statement* reports the operating performance over a short period of time, normally no less than one month and no more than one year. It shows revenues produced from operations and expenditures of monies used to generate those revenues (see Exhibit 1-3, *Income Statement*, p.83).

Normally, a medical practice is accounted for on the cash basis. This simply means that revenues are recognized when collected and expenses are recognized when paid. This does not negate the necessity to report total production within a practice or, differently stated, to report the total revenue from all sources for professional services. In today's health care environment, a significant portion of the production or revenue booked within a medical practice is never collected. Discounts are given to payors as contractual adjustments; governmental fee structures for Medicare and Medicaid patients reduce the amount collected. Nevertheless, the practice Income Statement, prepared on the cash basis, does not consider any revenue until the actual cash is received and deposited into the practice's bank account. Accounting on the cash basis does not mean that the practice would not maintain a separate accounts receivable ledger.

Bottom line results are expressed in the terminology *Net Profit After Taxes*. Depending on the legal structure of the practice, taxes may or may not have a bearing. If the practice is structured as a sole proprietorship, the taxes on the income from the practice are paid by the physician on his individual income tax return (Schedule C of Form 1040). If the practice is legally established as a Subchapter S Corporation or Limited Liability Company, the profits are passed through to the shareholders (or partners) to be reported and paid as individual, personal taxes. This is usually accounted for on a K-1 Form from the corporate or partnership tax return and reported on Schedule E of the individual's tax return. If the practice is established as a standard operating corporation, or better stated a "C" Corporation, it is subject to its own tax liability. Thus, the term *Net Profit After Taxes* is applicable. Usually, the profit or loss is transferred from profit and loss accounts to the retained earnings of the balance sheet's capital section. If a practice produces profit, the "net worth" in its capital account increases. Conversely, any loss reduces capital.

A *Balance Sheet* reflects the longer-term, general financial condition of the practice by showing specific assets versus liabilities of the practice. The net difference then is the capital or net worth of the practice. Many practices distribute all of their earnings to the physician(s). Thus, theoretically, there are no "retained earnings" or net worth on the Balance Sheet; all such earnings, past and current, are distributed. This does not mean that the practice has no value. The assets on the Balance Sheet have value to most purchasers of the practice. The possibility for an intangible or goodwill component of value also exists. However, it is not appropriate to recognize such value on the practice's Balance Sheet (see Exhibit 5-1, *Balance Sheet*, p.99).

Working Capital

Working capital is a very important component of operating a practice. It simply represents the difference between the current assets and the current liabilities. In the short run, usually a period up to one year, a practice's primary task is to properly manage expenses to generate sufficient production and cash income. This generates working capital or positive cash flow. Working capital is used to run the practice on a day-to-day basis and ultimately to pay the physician or owners. A comfortable margin of working capital allows the practice not only to meet its obligations, but to investigate other opportunities within their marketplace. This assures growth and future financial stability.

Cash flow is critical to any business. Since most medical practices are small businesses without a significant borrowing capacity or retained cash flow, it is important to manage so that at all times it is generating positive cash flow. This enables the practice to meet all of its day-to-day operations, including payroll. Opportunities for future practice expansion can also be explored.

CHAPTER 6

Reporting Practice Operating Results

The reporting process in today's operation of a medical practice is changing dramatically. As practices are being purchased by hospitals, independent operating companies, health maintenance organizations, and other investors, reporting must become more advanced, organized, and accurate. This holds true as well for the physician-owned and operated practices.

To provide management with adequate information, the reporting process must have the following characteristics:

- **Timeliness**
  Reflect recent historical results in reports.

- **Accuracy**
  Compile reliable and accurate data.

- **Simplicity**
  Provide information that is easy to interpret and understand. Rather than submitting reams of computer runs and various spread sheets of statistical data, keep reports simple and to the point.

- **Sufficiently Detailed**
  While keeping reports simple, include enough detail to provide sufficient data for making future decisions. Also detail only relevent amounts.

- **Quantitative**
  Use comparative analytical data from budgeted and prior period actual performance totals as a benchmark for measuring current operating performance.

- **Historical Data**
  Use historical data primarily as a basis for making future decisions.

The reporting cycle should be completed on a regular basis, at least quarterly and preferably monthly. Management will benefit by seeing operational results regularly, essentially at the same time each month. The process should be interpretive, with conclusions drawn and trends assessed. "Bullet points" can be used to concisely and simply interpret and summarize the data.

The reporting process should also be objective, depicting the true picture of the financial status of the practice. Both good and bad points should be included in the summary and in any conversation that occurs as reports are reviewed.

Finally, the information should be used to make informed decisions regarding the operations of the practice. In other words, it should be *reactive.* No physician or owner of a practice can simply take numbers on a page and fully understand the complete operations of the practice. The ability to make sound decisions increases when the information process includes concisely summarized reports with narrative interpretations, both written and verbal, and consultation between the practice administrator and physician.

Financial Analysis — Simplified

Medical practice management has become extraordinarily complex in recent years, leading many individuals to specialize in practice management as a career. In addition to physicians, highly proficient and competent specialists may be involved in the operations of a medical practice. The technical experts who assist in the operation and management of a practice may include a highly trained practice administrator and/or outside consultants. They may be prone to generate complicated financial analysis that is burdensome to interpret. To achieve the goals of providing operational information that prepares management to make sound business decisions, it is important to understand financial analysis and keep it simple.

What is Financial Analysis?

Financial analysis consists of the interpretation and evaluation of numerical relationships among figures in financial reports. For a medical practice, the most important financial report is its Income Statement *(the statement of revenues, expenses, gains, and losses for the period ending with net income for the period).* To a lesser extent, a Balance Sheet *(statement of financial position that shows Total Assets = Total Liabilities + Owners' Equity)* is also a key financial report. These two financial reports are interrelated. While most practices operate on a **cash basis** of accounting (i.e., revenue recognized when collected and expenses recognized when paid) the relationship between the Balance Sheet and Income Statement still exists. In *cash based* accounting, the Balance Sheet, showing accrual based items such as accounts receivable, accounts payable and accrued liabilities, is probably not as useful and functional when provided on a month-to-month basis.

Nevertheless, evaluating the meanings of key numbers on both the Income Statement and the Balance Sheet from one period to another gives management a basis for comparison. It distinguishes areas of the practice that are performing efficiently and profitably from problem areas that need to be addressed.

Through financial analysis the relationship between income, costs and cash flow is identified. Also, management (including the physician) can evaluate the financial health, leverage and deployment of assets and the working capital of the practice.

Financial Analysis Perspectives

Financial analysis is used by management for many purposes. Depending on the perspective, these purposes may include the following:

- Operational Control
- Pricing/Fee Structure
- Cost Evaluation
- Procurement of Capital (Financing)

- Measurement of Incremental Performance (e.g., departments within the practice)
- Profitability Analysis
- Return on Capital Analysis

These same principles are used in the analysis of all businesses. Traditionally, medical practices have not incorporated these analyses into their management. Yet now, as the health care environment has become more complex, with practices becoming larger and owned by various entities, financial analyses are essential to practice operation and management.

Whatever the analyst's point of view, financial viability must be interpreted in the following areas:

- Financial Health of the Practice
- Earning Potential of the Practice
- Liquidity of Assets
- Assessment of Risk

Each of these is critical in various forms: (1) to the existing owners of the practice; (2) as considerations for selling the practice; and, (3) to prospective, new owners reviewing the viability of it as an investment.

(See Exhibit 1-3, Income Statement, p.16, 83)
(See Exhibit 5-1, Balance Sheet, p.99)

CHAPTER 7

Financial Language Glossary

Since financial analysis and financial statement relationships include an understanding of not only the numbers that make up the reports, but also the terminologies, this chapter summarizes the ones that are pertinent to the medical practice.

Account Payable

A *liability* representing an amount owed to a *creditor*, usually arising from purchase of *merchandise* or materials and supplies; not necessarily due or past due. Normally, a current liability, arising from the day-to-day operation of the business.

Account Receivable

A claim against a *debtor* usually arising from sales or services rendered; not necessarily due or past due. Normally, a *current* asset, and arising from the normal course of business.

Accounting

A service activity whose function is to provide quantitative information, primarily financial in nature, about economic entities that is intended to be useful in making economic decisions.

Accounting Equation

Assets = Liabilities + Owners' Equity.

Accounting Period

The time period for which *financial statements* that measure *flows*, such as the *income statement* and the *statement of cash flows*, are prepared. Should be clearly defined on the financial statements. Normally, for no less than one month and no more than one year.

Accounting System

The procedures for collecting and summarizing financial data in a firm.

Accounts Receivable Turnover

Net *sales on account* divided by average *accounts receivable*. See ratio.

Accrual Basis of Accounting

The method of recognizing *revenues* as goods are sold (or delivered) and as services are rendered, independent of the time when cash is received. *Expenses* are recognized in the period when the related revenue is recognized independent of the time when cash is paid out.

Acquisition Cost

Of an *asset*, the net *invoice* price plus all *expenditures* to place and ready the asset for its intended use. The other expenditures might include legal fees, transportation charges, and installation costs.

Adjusted Bank Balance of Cash

The *balance* shown on the statement from the bank plus or minus amounts, such as for unrecorded deposits or outstanding checks, to reconcile the bank's balance with the correct cash balance.

Adjusted Book Balance of Cash

The *balance* shown in the firm's account for cash in bank plus or minus amounts, such as for *notes* collected by the bank or bank service charges, to reconcile the account balance with the correct cash balance.

Adjusting Entry

An entry made at the end of an *accounting period* to record a *transaction* or other *accounting event*, which for some reason has not been recorded or has been improperly recorded during the accounting period. An entry to update the accounts.

Administrative Expense

An *expense* related to the enterprise as a whole as contrasted to expenses related to more specific functions.

Admission of Partner

Legally, when a new partner joins a *partnership*, the old partnership is dissolved and a new one comes into being. In practice, however, the old accounting records may be kept in use and the accounting entries reflect the manner in which the new partnership joined the firm. If the new partner merely purchases the interest of another partner, the only accounting is to change the name for one capital account. If the new partner contributes *assets* and *liabilities* to the partnership, the new assets must be recognized with debits and the liabilities and other source of capital, with credits.

Aging Accounts Receivable

The process of classifying *accounts receivable* by the time elapsed since the claim came into existence for the purpose of estimating the amount of uncollectible accounts receivable as of a given date. It is also a management tool to determine wherein emphasis should be placed in order to complete collection of certain accounts receivable.

Allocate

To spread a *cost* from one *account* to several accounts, to several products, or activities, or to several periods, or to several cost centers. Would also apply to revenue in the same manner.

Americans with Disability Act (ADA)

The federal law that governs the rights of individuals with physical disabilities.

Amortization

The process of liquidating or extinguishing ("bringing of death") a *debt* with a series of payments to the *creditor* (or to a *sinking fund*.) From that usage has evolved a related use involving the accounting for the payments themselves: "amortization schedule" for a mortgage which is a table showing the allocation between *interest* and *principle*. The term has come to mean writing off ("liquidating") the cost of an asset. In this context, it means the general process of *allocating acquisition cost* of an asset to either the periods of benefit as *expenses* or to *inventory* accounts as *product costs*.

Appraisal

The process of obtaining a valuation for an *asset* or *liability* that involves expert opinion rather than evaluation of explicit market transactions.

Appreciation

An increase in economic worth caused by rising market prices for an asset.

Arm's Length

Said of a transaction negotiated by unrelated parties, each acting in his or her own self-interest; the basis for a *fair market value* determination.

Articles of Incorporation

Document filed with state authorities by persons forming a corporation. When the document is returned with a certificate of incorporation, it becomes the corporation's *charter*.

Assess

To value property for the purpose of property taxation; the assessment is computed by the taxing authority.

Asset

Defined as probable future economic benefits obtained or controlled by a particular entity as a result of past transactions.

Assignment of Accounts Receivable

Transfer of the legal ownership of an *account receivable* through its sale.

Audit

Systematic inspection of accounting records involving analyses, tests, and *confirmations*. See *internal audit*.

Bad Debt

An *uncollectible account* receivable.

Bad Debt Recovery

Collection, perhaps partial, of a specific account receivable previously written off an uncollectible.

Balance

As a noun, the sum of *debit* entries minus the sum of *credit* entries in an account.

Balance Sheet

Statement of financial position that shows *Total Assets* = Total Liabilities + Owners' Equity.

Balloon

Most *mortgage* and *installment loans* require relative equal periodic payments. Sometimes, the loan requires relatively equal periodic payments with a large final payment. The large final payment is called a "balloon" payment. Such loans are called "balloon" loans.

Bank Balance

The amount of the balance in a checking account shown on the *bank statement*.

Bank Reconciliation Schedule

A schedule that shows how the difference between the book balance of the cash in bank account and the bank's statement can be explained. Takes into account the amount of such items as checks issued that have not cleared or deposits that have not cleared or deposits that have not been recorded by the bank as well as errors made by the bank or the firm.

Bank Statement

A statement sent by the bank to a checking account customer showing deposits, checks cleared, and service charges for a period, usually one month.

Bankrupt

Said of a company whose *liabilities* exceed its assets where a legal petition has been filed and accepted under the bankruptcy law. A bankrupt firm is usually, but need not be, insolvent.

Bill

An *invoice* of charges and *terms of sale* for goods and services. Also, a piece of currency.

Bonus

Premium over normal *wage* or *salary*, paid usually for meritorious performance.

Book

As a verb, to record a transaction to the formal accounting records. As a noun, usually plural, the *journals* and *ledgers*. As an adjective, see *book value*.

Book Value

The amount shown in the books or in the accounts for an *asset, liability or owners' equity* item. Generally used to refer to the *net* amount of an *asset* or group of assets shown in the account which records the asset and reductions, such as for *amortization*, in its cost. Of a firm, the excess of total assets over total liabilities. *Net assets*.

Branch

A sales office or other unit of an enterprise physically separated from the home office of the enterprise but not organized as a legally separate *subsidiary*.

Breakeven Point

The volume of sales required so that total *revenues* and total *costs* are equal.

Budget

A financial plan that is used to estimate the results of future operations. Frequently used to control future operations.

Burn Rate

A new business usually begins life with cash-absorbing operating losses, but with a limited amount of cash. The "burn rate" measures how long the new business can survive before operating losses must stop or a new infusion of cash will be necessary. The measurement is ordinarily stated in terms of months.

Bylaws

The rules adopted by the shareholders of a corporation that specify the general methods for carrying out the functions of the corporation.

Capital

Owners' equity in a business. Often used, equally correctly, to mean the total assets of a business. Sometimes used to mean *capital assets*.

Capital Asset

Properly used, a designation for income tax purposes that describes property held by a taxpayer, except cash, inventorial assets, goods held primarily for sale, most depreciable property, *real estate*, *receivables*, certain *intangibles*, and a few other items.

Capital Budget

Plan of proposed outlays for acquiring long-term *assets* and the means of *financing* the acquisition.

Capital Gain

The excess of proceeds over *cost*, or other *basis*, from the sale of a *capital asset* as defined by the Internal Revenue Code. If the capital asset has been held for a sufficiently long time before sale, then the tax on the gain is computed at a rate lower than is used for other gains and ordinary income.

Capital Lease

A lease treated by the *lessee* as both the borrowing of funds and the acquisition of an asset to be *amortized*. Both the *liability* and the asset are recognized on the balance sheet. Expenses consist of *interest* on the *debt* and *amortization/depreciation* of the asset. The *lessor* treats the lease as the sale of the asset in return for a series of future cash receipts. Contrast with *operating lease*.

Capitalization of Earnings

The process of estimating the economic worth of a firm by computing the net present value of the predicted *net income* (not *cash flows*) of the firm for the future.

Cash

Currency and coins, negotiable checks, and balances in bank accounts. For the *statement of cash flows*, "cash" also includes *marketable securities* held as current assets.

Cash Basis of Accounting

In contrast to the *accrual basis of accounting*, a system of accounting in which *revenues* are recognized when cash is received and *expenses* are recognized as *disbursements* are made. No attempt is made to *match revenues* and *expenses* in determining *income*.

Cash Budget

A schedule of expected cash *receipts* and *disbursements*.

Cash Flow

Cash *receipts* minus *disbursements* from a given *asset*, or group of assets, for a given period.

Cash Receipts Journal

A specialized *journal* used to record all *receipts* of cash.

Certified Check

The check of a depositor drawn on a bank on the face of which the bank has inserted the words "accepted" or "certified" with the date and signature of a bank official. The check then becomes an obligation of the bank. Compares with *cashier's check*.

Chart of Accounts

A list of names and numbers, systematically organized, of *accounts*. It is from this basic listing that the General Ledger is formulated.

Check

The Federal Reserve Board defines a check as "a *draft* or order upon a bank or banking house purporting to be drawn upon a deposit of funds for the payment at all events of a certain sum of money to a certain person therein named or to him or his order or to bearer and payable instantly on demand." It must contain the phrase "pay to the order of." The amount shown on the check's face must be clearly readable and it must have the signature of the drawer. Checks need not be dated, although they usually are. The *balance* in the *cash account* is usually reduced when a check is issued, not later when it clears the bank and reduces cash in bank.

Check Register

A *journal* to record *checks* issued.

Close

As a verb, to transfer the balance of a *temporary* or *contra* or *adjunct* account to the main account to which it relates; for example, to transfer *revenue* and *expense* accounts directly, or through the *income summary*, to an *owners' equity* account, or to transfer *purchase discounts* to purchases. To "close" the books entails the above, usually done only once each year, at the end of the fiscal year.

Closing Entries

The *entries* that accomplish the transfer of balances in *temporary accounts* to the related *balance sheet accounts*.

Coinsurance

Insurance policies that project against hazards such as fire or water damage often specify that the owner of the property may not collect the full amount of insurance for a loss unless the insurance policy covers at least some specified "coinsurance" percentage, usually about 80 percent, of the *replacement cost* of the property. Coinsurance clauses induce the owner to carry full, or nearly full, coverage.

COLA

Cost-of-living adjustment. See *indexation*.

Collateral

Assets pledged by a *borrower* that will be given up if the *loan* is not paid.

Collectible

Capable of being converted into *cash*; now, if due; later, otherwise.

Commercial Paper

Short-term notes issued by corporate borrowers.

Commission

Remuneration, usually expressed as a percentage, to employees based upon an activity rate, such as sales.

Comparative (Financial) Statements

Financial statements showing information for the same company for different times, usually two successive years. Nearly all published financial statements are in this form. Contrast with *historical summary*.

Compound Interest

Interest calculated on *principal* plus previously undistributed interest.

Consolidated Financial Statements

Statements issued by legally separate companies but common ownership that show financial position and income as they would appear if the companies were one economic *entity*.

Control System

A device for ensuring that actions are carried out according to plan or for safeguarding *assets*. A system for ensuring that actions are carried out according to plan can be designed for a single function within the firm, called "operational control," for autonomous segments within the firm that generally have responsibility for both revenues and costs, called "divisional control," or for activities of the firm as a whole, called "company-wide control." Systems designed for safeguarding *assets* are called "internal control" systems.

Controller

The title often used for the chief accountant of an organization. Often spelled *comptroller*.

Corporation

A legal entity authorized by a state to operate under the rules of the entity's *charter*.

Correcting Entry

An *adjusting entry* where an improperly recorded *transaction* is properly recorded. Not to be confused with entries that correct *accounting errors*.

Cost

The sacrifice, measured by the *price* paid or required to be paid, to acquire *goods* or *services*.

Cost Center

A unit of activity for which *expenditures* and *expenses* are accumulated.

Credit

As a noun, an entry on the right-hand side of an account. As a verb, to make an entry on the right-hand side of an account. Records increases in *liabilities*, *owner's equity*, *revenues* and *gains*; records decreases in assets and expenses. See *debit and credit conventions*. Also the ability or right to buy or borrow in return for a promise to pay later.

Credit Memorandum

A document used by a seller to inform a buyer that the buyer's *account receivable* is being credited (reduced) because of *errors*, *returns*, or *allowances*. Also, the document provided by a bank to a depositor to indicate that the depositor's balance is being increased because of some event other than a deposit, such as the collection by the bank of the depositor's *note receivable*.

Current Asset

Cash and other *assets* that are expected to be turned into cash, sold, or exchanged within the normal operating cycle of the firm, usually one year. Current *assets* include *cash*, *marketable securities*, *receivable*, *inventory*, and *current prepayments*.

Current Funds

Cash and other assets readily convertible into cash.

Current Liability

A debt or other obligation that must be discharged within a short time, usually the *earnings cycle* or one year, normally by expending *current assets*.

Current Replacement Cost

Of an *asset*, the amount currently required to acquire an identical asset (in the same condition and with the same service potential) or an asset capable of rendering the same service at a current *fair market price*.

Customers' Ledger

The *ledger* that shows accounts receivable of individual customers. It is the *subsidiary ledger* for the *controlling account*, Accounts Receivable.

Debit

As a noun, an entry on the left hand side of an *account*. As a verb, to make an entry on the left hand side of an account. Records increases in *assets* and *expenses*; records decreases in *liabilities, owners' equity*, and *revenues*.

Debit Memorandum

A document used by a seller to inform a buyer that the seller is debiting (increasing) the amount of the buyer's *account receivable*. Also, the document provided by a bank to a depositor to indicate that the depositor's *balance* is being decreased because of some event other than payment for a *check*, such as monthly service charges or the printing of checks.

Debt

An amount owed. The general name for *notes, bonds, mortgages*, and the like that are evidence of amounts owed and have definite payment dates.

Deferral

The accounting process concerned with past *cash receipts* and *payments*; in contrast to *accrual*. Recognizing a liability resulting from a current cash receipt (as for magazines to be delivered) or recognizing an asset from a current cash payment (or for prepaid insurance or a long-term depreciable asset).

Defined Contribution Plan

A *money purchase (pension) plan* or other arrangement, based on formula or discretion, where the employer makes cash contributions to eligible individual employee *accounts* under the terms of a written plan document. Profit-sharing pension plans are of this type.

Depreciation

Amortization of plant assets; the process of allocating the cost of an asset to the periods of benefit — *the depreciable life*. Classified as a *production cost* or a *period expense*, depending upon the asset and whether *absorption* or *variable costing* is used.

Disbursement

Payment by *cash* or by *check*.

Double Entry

The system of recording transactions that maintains the equality of the accounting equation; each entry results in recording equal amounts of *debits* and *credits*.

Endorsement

See *draft*. The *payee* signs the draft and transfers it to a fourth party, such as the payee's bank.

Equity

A claim to *assets*; a source of assets.

ERISA

Employment Retirement Income Security Act of 1974. The federal law that sets most *pension plan* requirements.

Expense

As a noun, a decrease in *owners' equity* caused by the using up of *assets* in producing *revenue* or carrying out other activities that are part of the entity's *operations*.

Fair Market Price (Value)

Price (value) negotiated at *arm's-length* between a willing buyer and a willing seller, each acting rationally in his or her own self interest. May be estimated in the absence of a monetary transaction.

FICA

Federal Insurance Contributions Act. The law that sets *"Social Security" taxes* and benefits. Also includes Medicare taxes as a portion thereof.

Financial Projection

An estimate of *financial position*, results of *operations*, and changes in cash flows for one or more periods based on a set of assumptions. If the assumptions are not necessarily the most likely outcomes, then the estimate is called a "projection." If the assumptions represent the most probable outcomes, then the estimate is called a "forecast." "Most probable" means that the assumptions have been evaluated by management and that they are management's judgement of the most likely set of conditions and most likely outcomes. Statement of the *assets* and *equities* of a firm displayed as a *balance sheet*.

Financial Statements

The *balance sheet, income statement, statement of retained earnings, statement of cash flows, statement of retained earnings*, statement of changes of *owners' equity accounts*, and *notes* thereto.

Fiscal Year

A period of 12 consecutive months chosen by a business as the *accounting period* for annual reports. May or may not be a *natural business year* or a calendar year.

Fixed Cost (Expense)

An *expenditure* or *expense* that does not vary with volume of activity, at least in the short run.

Float

Checks whose amounts have been *added* to depositor's bank account, but not yet subtracted from the *drawer's* bank account.

Foreclosure

The borrower fails to make a required payment on a *mortgage*; the lender takes possession of the property for his or her use or sale. Assume that the lender sells the property but the proceeds of sale are insufficient to cover the outstanding balance on the loan at the time of foreclosure. Under the terms of most mortgages, the lender becomes an unsecured creditor of the borrower for the still-unrecovered balance of the loan.

Fully Vested

Said of a *pension plan* when an employee (or his or her estate) has rights to all the benefits purchased with the employer's contributions to the plan even if the employee is not employed by this employer at the time of death or retirement.

FUTA

Federal Unemployment Tax Act which provides for taxes to be collected at the federal level, to help subsidize the individual states' administration of their employment compensation programs.

General Journal

The formal record where transactions, or summaries of similar transactions, are recorded in *journal entry* form as they occur. Use of the adjective "general" usually implies only two columns for cash amounts or that there are also various *special journals*, such as a *check register*, or *sales journal*, in use.

General Ledger

The name for the formal *ledger* containing all of the financial statement accounts.

Goodwill

The excess of cost of an acquired firm (or operating unit) over the current *fair market value* of the separately identifiable *net assets* of the acquired unit. Before goodwill is recognized, all identifiable assets, whether or not on the books of the acquired unit, must be given a *fair market value*.

Grandfather Clause

An exemption in new accounting *pronouncements* exempting transactions that occurred before a given date from the new accounting treatment.

Gross

Not adjusted or reduced by deductions or subtractions. Contrast with *net*.

Holding Company

A company that confines its activities to owning *stock* in, and supervising management of, other companies. A holding company usually owns a controlling interest in, that is more than 50 percent of the voting stock of, the companies whose stock it holds.

Income

Excess of revenues and *gains* over *expenses* and *losses* for a period; *net income*. Sometimes used with an appropriate modifier to refer to the various intermediate amounts shown in a *multiple-step income statement*. Sometimes used to refer to revenues, as in "rental income."

Income Accounts

Revenue and *expense accounts*.

Income Statement

The statement of *revenues*, *expenses*, *gains*, and *losses* for the period ending with *net income* for the period.

Income Tax

An annual tax levied by the federal and other governments on the income of an entity.

Indexation

An attempt by lawmakers of parties to a contract to cope with the effects of *inflation*. Amounts fixed in law or contracts are "indexed" when these amounts change as a given measure of price changes.

Inflation

A time of generally rising prices.

Information System

A system, sometimes formal and sometimes informal, for collecting, processing and communicating data that are useful for the managerial functions of decision making, planning, and control, and for financial reporting.

Installment

Partial payment of a debt or collection of a receivable, usually according to a contract.

Insurance

A contract for reimbursement of specific losses, purchased with insurance premiums. Self-insurance is not insurance but merely the willingness to assume risk of incurring losses while saving the premium.

Intangible Asset

A nonphysical, *noncurrent* right that gives a firm an exclusive or preferred position in the marketplace. Examples are a *copyright*, *patent*, *trademark*, *goodwill*, *organization costs*, *capitalized* advertising costs, computer programs, licenses for any of the preceding, government licenses, *leases*, franchises, mailing lists, exploration permits, import and export permits, construction permits, and marketing quotas.

Interest

The charge or cost for using money; expressed as a rate per period, usually one year, called the "interest rate."

Internal Audit

An *audit* conducted by employees to ascertain whether or not *internal control* procedures are working, as opposed to an external audit conducted by a CPA.

Internal Revenue Service (IRS)

Agency of the U.S. Treasury Department responsible for administering the Internal Revenue Code and collecting income and certain other taxes.

In the Black (Red)

Operating at a profit (loss).

Inventory

As a noun, the *balance* in an asset *account* such as raw materials, supplies, work in process, and finished goods. As a verb, to calculate the *cost* of goods on hand at a given time or to physically count items on hand.

Investment

An *expenditure* to acquire property or other assets in order to produce *revenue*; the *asset* so acquired; hence a *current* expenditure made in anticipation of future income.

Journal

The place where transactions are recorded as they occur. The book of original entry.

Journal Entry

A recording in a *journal*, of equal *debits* and *credits*, with an explanation of the *transaction*, if necessary.

Kiting

This term means slightly different things in banking and auditing contexts. In both, however, it refers to the wrongful practice of taking advantage of the *float*, the time that elapses between the deposit of a *check* in one bank and its collection at another.

Lapping (accounts receivable)

The theft, by an employee, of cash sent in by a customer to discharge the latter's *payable*. The theft from the first customer is concealed by using cash received from a second customer. The theft from the second customer is concealed by using the cash received from a third customer, and so on. The process is continued until the thief returns the funds or can make the theft permanent by creating a fictitious *expense* or receivable write-off, or until the fraud is discovered.

Lease

A contract calling for the lessee (user) to pay the lessor (owner) for the use of an asset.

Leasehold Improvement

An *improvement* to leased property. Should be *amortized* over *service life* or the life of the lease, whichever is shorter.

Ledger

A book of accounts.

Liability

An obligation to pay a definite (or reasonably definite) amount at a definite (or reasonably definite) time in return for a past or current benefit. A liability has three essential characteristics: (1) an obligation to transfer assets or services at a specified or determinable date, (2) the entity has little or no discretion to avoid the transfer, and (3) the event causing the obligation has already happened; that is, is not executory.

Limited Partner

Member of a *partnership* not personally liable for debts of the partnership; every partnership must have at least one *general partner* who is fully liable.

Liquid Assets

Cash, current marketable securities, and sometime, *current receivables.*

Loan

An arrangement where the owner of property, called the lender, allows someone else, called the borrower, the use of the property for a period of time that is usually specified in the agreement setting up the loan. The borrower promises to return the property to the lender and, often, to make a payment for use of the property. Generally used when the property is *cash* and the payment for its use is *interest.*

Loss

Excess of cost over net proceeds for a single transaction; negative *income* for a period. A cost expiration that produced no *revenue.*

Margin

Revenue less specified expenses.

Merger

The joining of two or more businesses into a single *economic entity.* See *holding company.*

Mortgage

A claim given by the borrower (mortgage) against the borrower's property in return for a loan.

Negotiable

Legally capable of being transferred by endorsement. Usually said of *checks* and *notes* and sometimes of *stocks* and *bearer bonds.*

Net

Reduced by all relevant deductions.

Net Income

The excess of all *expenses* and *gains* for a period over all *expenses* and *losses* of the period.

Net Loss

The excess of all *expenses* and *losses* for a period over all *revenues* and *gains* of the period.

Nonprofit Corporation

An incorporated *entity*, such as a hospital, with owners who do not share in the earnings. It usually emphasizes providing services rather than maximizing income.

Note

An unconditional written promise by the maker (borrower) to pay a certain amount on demand or at a certain future time.

OASD(H)I

Old Age, Survivors, Disability, and (Hospital) Insurance.

Operating

An adjective used to refer to *revenue* and *expense* items relating to the company's main line(s) of business.

OSHA

Occupational Safety and Health Act. The federal law that governs working conditions in commerce and industry.

Out-of-Pocket

Said of an *expenditure* usually paid for with cash. An *incremental* cost.

Outstanding

Unpaid or uncollected. When said of a check, it means a check issued that did not clear the *drawer's* bank prior to the *bank statement* due.

Overdraft

A check written on a checking account that contains funds less than the amount of the check.

Overhead Costs

Any cost not directly associated with the production or sale of identifiable goods and services.

P & L

Profit and loss statement, *income statement.*

Partnership

Contractual arrangement between individuals to share resources and operations in a jointly run business.

Payable

Unpaid but not necessarily due or past due.

Payroll Taxes

Taxes levied because salaries or wages are paid; for example, *FICA* and unemployment compensation insurance taxes. Typically, the employer pays a portion and withholds part of the employee's wage fund.

Pension Fund

Fund, the assets of which are to be paid to retired, ex-employees, usually as a *life annuity*. Usually held by an independent trustee and thus is not an *asset* of the employer.

Pension Plan

Details or provisions of employer's contract with employees for paying retirement *annuities* or other benefits.

Petty Cash Fund

Currency and coins maintained for expenditures that are made with cash on hand.

Prime Rate

The rate for loans charged by commercial banks to their creditworthy customers.

Principal

An amount in which *interest* is charged or earned. The *face amount* of a *loan*. Also, the absent owner (principal) who hires the manager or accountant (agent) in a "principal-agent" relationship.

Prior-period Adjustment

A *debit* or *credit* made directly to *retained earnings* (that does not affect income for the period) to adjust earnings as calculated for prior periods.

Pro Forma Statements

Hypothetical statements. Financial statements as they would appear if some event, such as a *merger* or increased production and sales, had occurred or were to occur. Pro forma is often spelled as one word.

Profit Center

A unit of activity for which both *revenue* or *expenses* are accumulated; contrast with *cost center*.

Profit Sharing Plan

A *defined contribution plan*, where the employer contributes amounts based on net *income*.

Promissory Note

An unconditional written promise to pay a specified sum of money on demand or at a specified date.

Prorate

To *allocate* in proportion to some base.

Purchase Order

Document authorizing a seller deliver goods with payment to be made later.

Ratio

The number resulting when one number is divided by another. Ratios are generally used to assess aspects of profitability, solvency, and liquidity. The commonly used financial ratios are of three kinds: (1) those that summarize some aspect of *operations* for a period, usually a year, (2) those that summarize some aspect of *financial position* at a given moment — the moment for which a balance sheet has been prepared, and (3) those that relate some aspect of operations to some aspect of financial position.

Receipt

Acquisition of *cash*.

Rent

A charge for use of land, buildings, or other assets.

Retained Earnings

Net *income* over the life of a corporation less all *dividends* (including capitalization through *stock dividends*); *owners'. equity* less *contributed capital*.

Revenue

The increase in *owners' equity* caused by a service rendered or the sale of goods. The monetary measure of a service rendered.

Risk

A measure of a variability of the *return on investment*. For a given expected amount of return, most people prefer less risk to more risk. Therefore, in national markets, investments with more risk usually promise, or are expected to yield, a higher rate or return than investments with lower risk. Most people use "risk" and "uncertainty" as synonyms. In technical language, however, these terms have different meanings. "Risk" is used when the probabilities attached to the various outcomes are known, such as the probabilities of heads or tails in the flip of a fair coin. "Uncertainty" refers to an event where the probabilities of the outcomes, such as winning or losing a lawsuit, can only be estimated.

Risk Premium

Extra compensation paid to an employee or extra *interest* paid to a lender, over amounts usually considered normal, in return for their undertaking to engage in activities more risky than normal.

ROI

Return on investment, but usually used to refer to a single project and expressed as a ration; *income* divided by average *cost* of *assets* devoted to the project.

Salary

Compensation earned by manager, administration, professional, not based on an hourly rate. Contrast with *wage*.

Sale

A *revenue* transaction where *goods* or *services* are delivered to a customer in return for cash or a contractual obligation to pay.

Simple Interest

Interest calculated on *principal* where interest earned during periods before maturity of the loan is neither added to the principal nor paid to the lender. *Interest = principal x interest rate x time.* Seldom used in economic calculations except for periods less than one year; contrast with *compound interest*.

Social Security Taxes

Taxes levied by the federal government on both employers and employees to provide *funds* to pay retired persons (or their survivors) who are entitled to receive such payments, either because they paid Social Security taxes themselves or because the Congress has declared them eligible.

Sole Proprietorship

All *owners' equity* belongs to one person.

Spread Sheet

A *worksheet* organized like a *matrix* that provides a two-way classification of accounting data.

T-account

Account form shaped like the letter T with the title above the horizontal line. *Debits* are shown to the left of the vertical line, *credits* to the right.

Take-home Pay

The amount of a paycheck; earned wages or *salary* reduced by deductions for *income taxes*, *Social Security taxes*, contributions to fringe benefit plans, union dues, and so on.

Tax Credit

A subtraction from taxes otherwise payable, contrast with *tax deduction*.

Tax Deduction

A subtraction from *revenues* and *gains* to arrive at taxable income. Tax deductions are technically different from tax *exemptions*, but the effect of both is to reduce gross income in computing taxable income. Both are different from *tax credits*, which are subtracted.

Taxable Income

Income computed according to IRS regulation and subject to *income taxes*. Contrast with income, net income, income before taxes (in the *income statement*), and *comprehensive income* (a *financial reporting* concept). Use the term "pretax income" to refer to income before taxes on the income statement in financial reports.

Tickler File

A collection of *vouchers* or other memoranda arranged chronologically to remind the person in charge of certain duties to make payments (or to do other tasks) as scheduled.

Trial Balance

A listing of *account balances*: all accounts with *debit* balances are totaled separately from accounts with *credit* balances. The two totals should be equal. Trial balances are taken as a partial check of the arithmetic accuracy of the entries previously made.

Underwriter

One who agrees to purchase an entire *security issue* for a specified price, usually for resale to others.

Value

Monetary worth; the term is usually so subjective that it ought not to be used without a modifying adjective unless most people would agree on the amount; not to be confused with cost. See *fair market value*.

Variance

Difference between actual and *standard costs* or between *budgeted* and actual *expenditures* or, sometimes, *expenses*.

Vendor

A seller.

Value

Monetary worth; the term is usually so subjective that it ought not to be used without a modifying adjective unless most people would agree on the amount; not to be confused with cost. See *fair market value*.

Vested

Said of an employee's *pension plan* benefits that are not contingent on the employee's continuing to work for the employer.

Wage

Compensation of employees based on time worked or output of product for manual labor. See *take-home pay*.

Warranty

A promise by a seller to correct deficiencies in products sold.

Weighted Average

An average computed by counting each occurence of each value, not merely a single occurence of each value.

Withdrawals

Assets distributed to an owner.

Withholding

Deductions from *salaries* or *wages*, usually for *income taxes*, to be remitted by the employer, in the employee's name, to the taxing authority.

Write Down

Write off, except that not all of the asset's cost is charge to expense or *loss*. Generally used for nonrecurring items.

Write Off

Charge an asset to *expense* or *loss*; that is, *debit* expense (or loss) and *credit* asset.

Exhibits

Budget Planning Worksheet

Exhibit 1-1-1

Items	1993	1994	% Change	1995	% Change	Initial Budget	Final Budget	% of Revenue
Revenue "Net Collections"*								
Accounting/Legal								
Contributions								
Dues/Subscriptions								
Equipment Rental								
General Insurance								
Health Insurance								
Malpractice Insurance								
Lab Fees								
Janitorial								
Medical Supplies								
Office Supplies								
Rent or Lease								
Salaries								
Taxes-Payroll								
Taxes-Other								
Telephone								
Postage								
Maintenance, Repairs								
Interest								
Depreciation								
Professional Services								
Profit Sharing								
Other								
Total Expenses								
Net Income Pre-Physician Comp.								

Patient Cost Analysis

Exhibit 1-2-1

1. Total number of patients seen for prior 12 months .... _____

2. Total of all expenses for prior 12 months .... _____

3. Subtract from line 2 all **Fixed Expenses** (rent, salaries
   and benefits, insurance, utilities) .... _____

4. Total **Patient** expenses for prior 12 months... _____

5. Total receipts for prior 12 months.. _____

6. Divide line 5 by line 1 to get gross revenue per patient... _____

7. Divide line 4 by line 1 to get cost per patient... _____

8. Subtract line 7 from line 6 to get revenue per patient .... _____

Income Statement

Exhibit 1-3

	Current Month			Year-to-date		
	Budget	**Actual**	**% Variance**	**Budget**	**Actual**	**% Variance**
Income						
Charges						
Other Adjustments						
Other Receipts						
Total Income						
Expenses						
Salaries – Office						
Answering Service and Pager						
Automobile						
Consultant Fees						
Conventions and Meetings						
Contributions						
Depreciation						
Dues/Subscriptions						
Employee Benefits						
Gifts/Flowers						
Insurance – Business						
Insurance – Malpractice						
Laundry – Uniforms						
Legal & Accounting						
Medical Pamphlets & Books						
Miscellaneous						
Office Supplies & Expense						
Postage						
Profit Sharing						
Rent						
Repairs & Maintenance						
Supplies – Medical						
Taxes & Licenses						
Telephone						
Transcription Fees						
X-Ray Expense						
Total Expenses						
Operating Income <Loss>						

REVENUE/COST ANALYSIS FOR _____

Revenues $_____

Direct Cost

    Salary/Benefits [1] $_____

    Cost of Supplies $_____

    Supplies [2] $_____

    Equipment Depreciation [3] $_____

    Maintenance & Repairs $_____

    Total Direct Costs $_____

    Contribution Margin $_____

Indirect Costs

    Building Lease [4] $_____

    Utilities $_____

    Miscellaneous [5] $_____

    Total Direct Costs $_____

    Division Profit $_____

---

[1] Based on 80% of one employee's time.

[2] Based on $_____ per test.

[3] Based on _____ year life expectancy.

[4] Costs in this category are based on the proportion of square footage occupied by the equipment, if applicable.

[5] Janitorial, laundry, maintenance, property tax.

Service	Current Fee	Cost of Supplies Needed	Net Profit

	Goal	Current Month	Previous Month	YTD
Billings				
Collections				
Adjustments				
Collections Percentage (Fee-for-service cash collections ÷ Gross fee-for-service charges)				
Total Accounts Receivable				
Accounts Receivable Ratio (Total Accounts Receivable ÷ Average monthly billings)				
New Patients				
Total Patient Visits				
Expense Ratio (Total non-physician expense ÷ Total gross charges)				
Profit <Loss> (Collections minus expenses)				
Net Income Percentage (Total net income ÷ collections)				

Month: _____

Total Charges: .... _____

Adjustments: .... _____

Net Charges: .... _____

Total Receipts: .... _____

Adjustments: .... _____

Net Receipts: .... _____

Total Patients Seen: .... _____

Daily Average: .... _____

Collection Ratio: .... _____

Accounts Receivable: .... _____

Average Per Patient Charge: .... _____

Average Per Patient Cost: .... _____

Total Monthly Expense: .... _____

Net Income: .... _____

Disbursements		Date Starting: _____ Date Ending: _____		
		(A) Starting Balance $_____		
No.	**Date**	**Item Purchased**	**(B) Amount**	**(C) Balance**
			Total	

Total Transactions: (A)   –   (B)   =   (C)

$ _____ $ _____ $ _____

Request for Reimbursement: $ _____

Submitted By: _____ Date: _____

Mail Receipts Journal			Reciepts as of: _____	
Check/Reference Number, etc.	**Source**	**Sender**	**City/State**	**Amount**
			Total	

Prepared By:_____   Date:_____

Daily Collections Summary

Exhibit 4-3

Date: _____

Check No.	Description/ Patient Name	Physician	Cash	Check	Credit Card	Total	Payment Received

Balance Sheet (Example)

Exhibit 5-1

Central Medical Associates
Statement of Assets, Liabilities, and Equity
as of December 31, 19___.

ASSETS

Current Assets

Petty Cash	$	125
Primary Care Operations Account		9,499
Primary Care Cash Receipts Account		120
Total Current Assets		**$ 9,744**

Property and Equipment

Office Equipment	$	30,031
Accumulated Depreciation – Office Equipment		(26,832)
Medical Equipment		59,022
Accumulated Depreciation – Medical Equipment		(58,097)
Furniture and Fixtures		7,080
Accumulated Depreciation – Furniture and Fixtures		(7,080)
Intangible Assets (software)		995
Accumulated Amortization – Intangible Assets (software)		(596)
Leasehold Improvements		9,792
Accumulated Amortization – Leasehold Improvements		(5,809)
Total Property and Equipment		**8,506**

Other Assets

Deposits	$	890
Total Other Assets		**890**
Total Assets		***$19,140***

LIABILITIES AND STOCKHOLDER'S EQUITY

Current Liabilities

Payroll Taxes Payable	$	856
Note Payable – Bank (due within one year)		10,500
Total Current Liabilities		**$11,356**
Total Liabilities		***$11,356***

Stockholder's Equity

Capital Stock	$	2,775
Retained Earnings		(6,375)
Net Income (Loss) – Y-T-D		(3,898)
Accumulated Adjustments Account (Sub S-Corp.)		15,282
Total Stockholder's Equity		**$7,784**
Total Liabilities and Equity		***$19,140***

Balance Sheet

Exhibit 5-1

Practice Name: _____

ASSETS

Statement of Assets, Liabilities, and Equity
as of (date): ____ / ____ / ____ .

Current Assets

Petty Cash .... $ _____
Primary Care Operations Account .... _____
Primary Care Cash Receipts Account............................. _____

Total Current Assets.. $ _____

Property and Equipment

Office Equipment.. $ _____
Accumulated Depreciation – Office Equipment .... _____
Medical Equipment... _____
Accumulated Depreciation – Medical Equipment .... _____
Furniture and Fixtures... _____
Accumulated Depreciation – Furniture and Fixtures .... _____
Intangible Assets (software) .... _____
Accumulated Amortization – Intangible Assets (software)............. _____
Leasehold Improvements... _____
Accumulated Amortization – Leasehold Improvements .... _____

Total Property and Equipment .... $ _____

Other Assets

Deposits .... $ _____

Total Other Assets.. $ _____

Total Assets... $ _____

LIABILITIES AND STOCKHOLDER'S EQUITY

Current Liabilities

Payroll Taxes Payable ....$ _____
Note Payable – Bank (due within one year)................... _____

Total Current Liabilities .... $ _____

Total Liabilities... $ _____

Stockholder's Equity

Capital Stock ....$ _____
Retained Earnings .... _____
Net Income (Loss) – Y-T-D .... _____
Accumulated Adjustments Account (Sub S-Corp.) .... _____

Total Stockholder's Equity .... $ _____

Total Liabilities and Equity .... $ _____

Index